ADAPTATION
THROUGH
OCCUPATION
MULTIDIMENSIONAL PERSPECTIVES

ADAPTATION
THROUGH
OCCUPATION
MULTIDIMENSIONAL PERSPECTIVES

Editors

Lenin C. Grajo, PhD, EdM, OTR/L
Director, Post-Professional
Doctor of Occupational Therapy (OTD) Program
Assistant Professor, Programs in Occupational Therapy
Department of Rehabilitation and Regenerative Medicine
Vagelos College of Physicians and Surgeons
Columbia University
New York, NY

Angela K. Boisselle, PhD, OTR, ATP
Utilization Management Therapy Supervisor
Cook Children's Health Care System
Fort Worth, TX

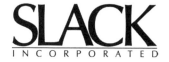

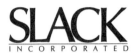

SLACK Incorporated
6900 Grove Road
Thorofare, NJ 08086 USA
856-848-1000   Fax: 856-848-6091
www.Healio.com/books
© 2019 by SLACK Incorporated

Senior Vice President: Stephanie Arasim Portnoy
Vice President, Editorial: Jennifer Kilpatrick
Vice President, Marketing: Michelle Gatt
Acquisitions Editor: Brien Cummings
Managing Editor: Allegra Tiver
Creative Director: Thomas Cavallaro
Cover Artist: Katherine Christie
Project Editor: Joseph Lowery

Adaptation Through Occupation: Multidimensional Perspectives includes ancillary materials specifically available for faculty use. Included are PowerPoint slides. Please visit http://www.efacultylounge.com to obtain access.

The procedures and practices described in this publication should be implemented in a manner consistent with the professional standards set for the circumstances that apply in each specific situation. Every effort has been made to confirm the accuracy of the information presented and to correctly relate generally accepted practices. The authors, editors, and publisher cannot accept responsibility for errors or exclusions or for the outcome of the material presented herein. There is no expressed or implied warranty of this book or information imparted by it. Care has been taken to ensure that drug selection and dosages are in accordance with currently accepted/recommended practice. Off-label uses of drugs may be discussed. Due to continuing research, changes in government policy and regulations, and various effects of drug reactions and interactions, it is recommended that the reader carefully review all materials and literature provided for each drug, especially those that are new or not frequently used. Some drugs or devices in this publication have clearance for use in a restricted research setting by the Food and Drug and Administration or FDA. Each professional should determine the FDA status of any drug or device prior to use in their practice.

Any review or mention of specific companies or products is not intended as an endorsement by the author or publisher.

SLACK Incorporated uses a review process to evaluate submitted material. Prior to publication, educators or clinicians provide important feedback on the content that we publish. We welcome feedback on this work.

Library of Congress Cataloging-in-Publication Data

Names: Grajo, Lenin C., editor. | Boisselle, Angela K., editor.
Title: Adaptation through occupation : multidimensional perspectives /
   [edited by] Lenin C. Grajo, Angela K. Boisselle.
Description: Thorofare, NJ : SLACK Incorporated, [2019] | Includes
   bibliographical references and index.
Identifiers: LCCN 2018031404 (print) | LCCN 2018032266 (ebook) | ISBN
   9781630914004 (Epub) | ISBN 9781630914011 (Web) | ISBN 9781630913991
   (paperback : alk. paper)
Subjects: | MESH: Occupational Therapy--methods | Adaptation, Physiological |
   Adaptation, Psychological | Occupational Health
Classification: LCC RM735.3 (ebook) | LCC RM735.3 (print) | NLM WB 555 | DDC
   615.8/515--dc23
LC record available at https://lccn.loc.gov/2018031404

Printed in the United States of America.

Last digit is print number: 10   9   8   7   6   5   4   3   2   1

DEDICATION

This book is especially dedicated to:

The leaders of the occupational therapy profession and occupational science who have helped create the construct of "adaptation through engagement in occupations."

All current educators, scholars, practitioners of occupational therapy, and occupational scientists who continue to apply the construct of occupational adaptation in teaching, practice, and research.

And to all current students—future practitioners and scholars—who dedicate themselves to building on the legacy and continuing to develop the body of knowledge on occupational adaptation.

CONTENTS

Dedication . . . .*v*

Acknowledgments . . . . *ix*

About the Editors . . . . *xi*

Contributing Authors . . . . *xiii*

Foreword by Sally W. Schultz, PhD, OT, LPC-S . . . . *xv*

Introduction . . . . *xix*

Section I	**Conceptual Evolution of Occupational Adaptation**

Overview. 1
Angela K. Boisselle, PhD, OTR, ATP
Lenin C. Grajo, PhD, EdM, OTR/L

Chapter 1 Defining the Construct of Occupational Adaptation 3
Lenin C. Grajo, PhD, EdM, OTR/L
Angela K. Boisselle, PhD, OTR, ATP
Elaina DaLomba, PhD, MSW, OTR/L

Chapter 2 Adaptation as a Measure of Occupational Participation 19
Lorrie George-Paschal, PhD, OTR/L, ATP
Lenin C. Grajo, PhD, EdM, OTR/L

Section II **Neuroscience Perspectives on Occupational Adaptation**
Overview. 33
Angela K. Boisselle, PhD, OTR, ATP
Lenin C. Grajo, PhD, EdM, OTR/L

Chapter 3 Neural Basis of Adaptation:
Neuroplasticity and Movement Sciences. 35
Dawn M. Nilsen, EdD, OTR/L, FAOTA
Angela K. Boisselle, PhD, OTR, ATP

Chapter 4 Neural Basis of Adaptation:
Motivation, Intention, Resilience, and
Goal-Directed Behaviors. 59
Katherine Dimitropoulou, PhD, OTR
Mary Frances Baxter, PhD, OT, FAOTA

Section III **Occupational Adaptation in**
Occupational Therapy Theories and Models
Overview. 81
Lenin C. Grajo, PhD, EdM, OTR/L
Angela K. Boisselle, PhD, OTR, ATP

Chapter 5   Occupational Adaptation as a Normative and
                 Intervention Process: New Perspectives on
                 Schkade and Schultz's Professional Legacy.................. 83
                 Lenin C. Grajo, PhD, EdM, OTR/L

Chapter 6   Formation of Identity and Occupational Competence:
                 Occupational Adaptation in the
                 Model of Human Occupation 105
                 Patricia Bowyer, EdD, MS, OTR, FAOTA

Chapter 7   Adaptation From a Sensory Processing Perspective........... 123
                 Lauren Little, PhD, OTR/L
                 Winifred Dunn, PhD, OTR, FAOTA

Chapter 8   Adaptation as a Transaction With the Environment:
                 Perspectives From the Ecology of
                 Human Performance Model...........................141
                 Evan E. Dean, PhD, OTR
                 Anna Wallisch, PhD, OTR/L
                 Winifred Dunn, PhD, OTR, FAOTA

Section IV   Occupational Adaptation in Occupational Science
                 Overview...157
                 Lenin C. Grajo, PhD, EdM, OTR/L
                 Angela K. Boisselle, PhD, OTR, ATP

Chapter 9   An Occupational Science Perspective on
                 Occupation, Adaptation, and Participation 159
                 Rebecca M. Aldrich, PhD, OTR/L
                 Kendra Heatwole Shank, PhD, OTR/L

Chapter 10   The Lived Experience of Occupational Adaptation:
                 Adaptation in the Wake of Adversity,
                 Life Transitions, and Change 175
                 Mandy Stanley, PhD

Financial Disclosures.......................................*193*
Index *195*

Acknowledgments

We both would like to thank Dr. Sally Schultz who has been one of the most inspiring mentors we have had in our careers. She has taught us to think critically, creatively, and reflectively throughout our doctoral journey and as scholars in the field. She has encouraged us to challenge paradigms, assert our voices, and gave us the "blessing" to expand on the work on occupational adaptation.

We would like to thank our contributing authors who have gone through this exciting journey with us. These authors are emerging and established scholars and leaders in occupational therapy and occupational science. They shared with us our vision for the book and our aim of advancing the body of knowledge on occupational adaptation.

We would like to thank our colleagues and friends at SLACK, Incorporated: Brien Cummings, our Acquisitions Editor; Allegra Tiver, our Managing Editor; and Joe Lowery, our Project Editor. Thank you for your guidance, your patience, your creativity, and for allowing us to develop and publish this text.

Notes of Gratitude from Dr. Lenin C. Grajo:

Thank you to my colleagues and mentors in the Programs in Occupational Therapy at Columbia University Irving Medical Center: Dr. Janet Falk-Kessler and Dr. Glen Gillen for your support and encouragement in this entire process; and especially to Dr. Sharon Gutman for your inspiration, mentorship, and friendship.

Thank you to Dr. Catherine Candler, my Texas Woman's University mentor, and Prof. Maria Concepcion Cabatan, my mentor from the University of the Philippines. Thank you for believing in me, allowing me to explore my intellectual curiosity, and providing me countless opportunities for professional growth.

Thank you to my aunt Elnora and my sister Marijo for your love and unwavering support.

Lastly, I want to thank all my former and current students, and all the children and families I have worked with as a practitioner. I cherish every memory and encounter and I owe so much of my personal and professional growth because you have allowed me to be a part of your lives.

Notes of Gratitude from Dr. Angela K. Boisselle:

Thank you to all of the children and families with whom I have worked over the years. It is from you that I learned the true meaning of resilience, strength, creativity, determination, compassion, and adaptation. You have taught me far more than I ever taught you.

Drs. Richard Adams, Mauricio Delgado, and Veronica Meneses from Texas Scottish Rite Hospital for Children. You not only enthusiastically share your knowledge about Pediatrics and Neuroscience, but also your passion for treating the whole child.

Drs. Mary Law, Peter Rosenbaum, and Iona Novak and Sue Baptiste. Your significant contributions to multidisciplinary research and scholarly work on cerebral palsy, participation, child-family engagement, and international practice, has made a tremendous impact on my career.

Above all, I would like to thank my daughters—my everything, Aliya and Marlee; my parents who taught me about hard work, stubbornness, and how to think differently; my sisters, you are my foundation; and my dear friend Jody who continues to keep me balanced with fun and laughter when I need it the most.

About the Editors

Lenin C. Grajo, PhD, EdM, OTR/L, is Assistant Professor of Rehabilitation and Regenerative Medicine (Occupational Therapy) in the Programs in Occupational Therapy at Columbia University Irving Medical Center in New York, NY. A pediatric occupational therapist by practice, he is a strong advocate of evidence-informed, occupation-based, theory-guided, client-centered, and occupational justice–promoting occupational therapy service provision.

Dr. Grajo is elected Chairperson of the Education Special Interest Section of the American Occupational Therapy Association (AOTA) and a voting member of the Commission on Education of AOTA from 2016-2019. He is a multi-awarded educator who has taught in the Philippines and the United States.

Angela K. Boisselle, PhD, OTR, ATP, has 18 years' experience as a pediatric occupational therapist and assistive technologist. She currently works at Cook Children's Health Plan as the Therapy Supervisor of Utilization Management. Her practice and research background include pediatric complex care, occupational adaptation, neuromuscular diseases, creativity, international occupational therapy, and assistive technology.

Dr. Boisselle is active with the American Academy of Cerebral Palsy and Developmental Medicine (AACPDM) and World Health Organization Global Cooperative on Assistive Technology (GATE). Dr. Boisselle has also served as a research consultant with University of Texas at Arlington Computer Science and Engineering Department since 2009. She has collaborated on several projects, including robotics, human computer interaction, and virtual rehabilitation.

CONTRIBUTING AUTHORS

Rebecca M. Aldrich, PhD, OTR/L (Chapter 9)
Associate Professor
USC Chan Division of Occupational Science and Occupational Therapy
University of Southern California
Los Angeles, California

Mary Frances Baxter, PhD, OT, FAOTA (Chapter 4)
Professor
School of Occupational Therapy
Texas Woman's University
Houston, Texas

Patricia Bowyer, EdD, MS, OTR, FAOTA, SFHEA (Chapter 6)
Professor and Doctoral Programs Coordinator
School of Occupational Therapy
Texas Woman's University
Houston, Texas

Elaina DaLomba, PhD, MSW, OTR/L (Chapter 1)
Assistant Professor
Occupational Therapy Department
Samuel Merritt University
Oakland, California

Evan E. Dean, PhD, OTR (Chapter 8)
Assistant Professor
Department of Occupational Therapy Education
Research Associate, Beach Center on Disability
Kansas University Center on Developmental Disabilities
University of Kansas Medical Center
Kansas City, Kansas

Katherine Dimitropoulou, PhD, OTR (Chapter 4)
Assistant Professor, Programs in Occupational Therapy
Department of Rehabilitation and Regenerative Medicine
Vagelos College of Physicians and Surgeons
Columbia University
New York, NY

Winifred Dunn, PhD, OTR, FAOTA (Chapters 7 & 8)
Distinguished Professor
Department of Occupational Therapy
University of Missouri
Columbia, Missouri

Lorrie George-Paschal, PhD, OTR/L, ATP (Chapter 2)
Professor
Department of Occupational Therapy
University of Central Arkansas
Conway, Arkansas

Kendra Heatwole Shank, PhD, OTR/L (Chapter 9)
Assistant Professor
Department of Occupational Therapy and Occupational Science
Towson University
Towson, Maryland

Lauren Little, PhD, OTR/L (Chapter 7)
Assistant Professor
Department of Occupational Therapy
Rush University
Chicago, Illinois

Dawn M. Nilsen, EdD, OTR/L, FAOTA (Chapter 3)
Associate Professor, Programs in Occupational Therapy
Department of Rehabilitation and Regenerative Medicine
Vagelos College of Physicians and Surgeons
Columbia University
New York, NY

Mandy Stanley, PhD (Chapter 10)
Associate Professor
School of Medical and Health Sciences
Edith Cowan University
Joondalup, Australia

Anna Wallisch, PhD, OTR/L (Chapter 8)
Postdoctoral Researcher
Juniper Gardens Children's Project
University of Kansas
Kansas City, Kansas

FOREWORD

The assembly of chapters in this scholarly work presents a set of timely perspectives that challenge the reader to examine his or her understanding of what is meant by the construct of occupational adaptation. As one of the original authors on Occupational Adaptation (OA) as a model for practice, I find that the combined works in this text offer an expanded and more integrated view on this construct. I had the pleasure of teaching OA to both of this text's editors. I made it very clear that it was my full intention to indoctrinate them into the world of OA. I quietly rejoiced in how spirited they were in challenging my efforts! I used a lot of stories and personal examples in class. Janette Schkade and I had just begun our work on OA when my son was born. I was in the kitchen, starting dinner, and looked down to watch him in the carrier with discovery toys hanging down. I noticed his eyes focused on the toys, an arm flailing around trying to get one. Suddenly, he actually touched it and the toy moved. A look of great surprise came over him, he thought for a few seconds, and then the arm went straight up and hit the toy. He was thrilled with delight, no doubt at his own pivotal experience of mastery over his environment. It was empowering. He had reorganized his *adaptation gestalt* and taken charge of his world. His sense of *relative mastery* was extremely high. My daughter was born before Janette and I developed the OA model. At about 18 months old, she was stacking a tower of wooden blocks. I went over to help her by showing how to straighten it so she could build higher. She glared at me, knocked it down, and stormed off. Years later, I realized it wasn't just that she didn't want me to help out; the issue was that I had interfered with her desire to master her environment and gain that sense of mastery for herself.

It is rewarding to see how the editors of this text have built upon their own relative mastery. They have enlightened the construct of occupational adaptation and added new dimensions to it. The text presents a masterful collection of writings that gives synergy to the overarching notions. They elegantly cajole the reader to examine his or her personal perspectives on the practice of occupational therapy—what it is, what we want it to be—and challenge those interested in this inquiry to step in and actively participate in shaping practice.

I suggest that the relationship between occupation and adaptation, and the construct of occupational adaptation, are prizes that the profession hasn't quite yet fully discovered. The literature and professional association tout occupation as the core value of the profession. Numerous professional publications cite occupation as both the means and the end of therapy. A number of scholars have also identified the ambiguity of this notion and recognized the need for clarity. This calls on the writer to share an example. Janette and I were definitely polar opposites. Her doctorate was in experimental psychology; my doctorate was in special education with children with emotional-behavior disorders. She practiced in orthopedics; I practiced in psychiatry. There was much we had to resolve in building our initial understanding of OA. A few years later, the PhD students began presenting their work at a biannual symposium at Texas Woman's University (TWU). Faculty also presented. Janette and I provided an update on OA. As I was concluding our presentation, I commented that occupation is the means and the individual's ability to adapt is the end. Janette snapped, "What! No, that's not true; occupation is the means and end!" There we were, in the thick of it, right in front of everyone. Janette retired a few years later. We didn't ever reach agreement. At last, I had the upper hand! Just to clarify, the point is that she and I had *never had* the discussion on our understanding of the means and end of occupational therapy. I suggest this discussion is one of the elephants in the room. The bigger elephant in the room should certainly be the relative absence of authentic occupation in practice. It is exciting to hear the various voices that speak to the reader in this text. Each chapter helps bring these issues into focus. Examining the means and end along with the construct of occupational adaptation could bring more clarity to who we are and who we want to be. The following quote speaks to this:

> *For last year's words belong to last year's language*
> *And next year's words await another voice.*
> — T. S. Eliot, *Four Quartets*

I propose that gaining greater clarity will require a more clearly defined common language of practice. Although "naming and framing" is powerful, it is not enough to provide the guideposts necessary to identify how to exemplify the importance of authentic occupation in everyday practice, along with the practice-based research needed to build evidence-based practice. The expected rigor lies within a common language that is not only consistent with the profession's philosophy and theoretically sound but is most importantly a common language that resonates with actual practice. Embracing occupation and adaptation and the construct of occupational adaptation across practice arenas, education, and research offers the profession an opportunity for increased depth, scope, and understanding in the means and end of occupational therapy.

While working at TWU, I frequently addressed laypersons attending occupational therapy events and fundraisers. I made it a point to say that, "Yes, indeed, occupational therapy can help people find or get back to their job; it might be an easy return after a knee replacement or therapy may be more complicated, and the individual may not be able to return to his or her previous job. But the goal of therapy will be about helping that person re-engage with the occupations of daily life that are personally meaningful. The person may need to learn how to do things differently, become more adaptive, and figure out how to do the desired occupations." I suggest that both the professional associations and educational programs will be key to promoting a paradigm shift that embraces the relationship between occupation and adaptation. The focus on an individual's ability to participate in an occupation is incomplete. There is more to being therapeutic. As part of rethinking the notion of means and end, it is essential to recapture the profession's perspective on therapeutic use of self in practice. Based on my observation and experience, it seems this has been lost. Practice appears to have acquired a primarily *a-priori* assumption; that is, if the therapist teaches the individual the skills needed to be functional, then he or she will be able to adapt. The construct of occupational adaptation is based on the contrary assumption that if the therapist works with the individual in a therapeutic relationship, focuses on helping the individual become as adaptive as possible, and functions as the agent of change, the individual will maximize his or her potential to function.

The collection of writings in this text makes a significant contribution to the body of knowledge in occupational therapy. They offer depth, insight, and integrated thinking that can facilitate the profession toward a more comprehensive understanding of therapy. They present the far-reaching significance of neuroscience in all practice arenas and a cogent argument for the need to reframe how the profession understands therapy, the process of the therapist being therapeutic, theoretical concepts, and the desired therapy outcomes. This text presents the merits of the profession embracing a broader understanding of the relationship between occupation and adaptation, as well as an examination of how the construct of occupational adaption may serve as a base to reintegrate therapeutic use of self, the power of authentic occupation, and the impact that promoting the individual's adaptiveness can have on treatment outcomes.

I close this Foreword with great hopes for the future of occupational therapy and its impact on individuals' lives. Occupational therapy is in good hands. The following is probably the most frequently published quotation in occupational therapy literature. I can't think of words that say it better:

> *We shall not cease from exploration*
> *And the end of all our exploring*
> *Will be to arrive where we started*
> *And know the place for the first time.*
> — T. S. Eliot, *Four Quartets*

Sally W. Schultz, PhD, OT, LPC-S
Professor Emerita
School of Occupational Therapy
Texas Woman's University
Proponent, Occupational Adaptation Model

INTRODUCTION

A Challenge to Use and Articulate the Construct of Occupational Adaptation

Occupations are activities that bring meaning to the daily lives of individuals, families, communities, and populations, and enable them to participate in society. All individuals have an innate need and right to engage in meaningful occupations throughout their lives. Participation in these occupations influences their development, health, and well-being across the life span. As such, participation in meaningful occupation is a determinant of health and leads to adaptation.
— *Philosophical Base of Occupational Therapy* (American Occupational Therapy Association, 2017)

The construct of *adaptation through occupation* is deeply grounded in the philosophical and historical roots of the profession. Adaptation is the mechanism by which person-environment-occupation transactions are manifested (Schultz & Schkade, 1997). Adolf Meyer (1922/1977) asserted that occupation is the primary means to positively influence man's ability to adapt. Yerxa (1992) eloquently stated that "the person is active, capable, free, self-directed, integrated, purposeful, and an agent who is the author of health-influencing activity" (p. 79). We view these foundational viewpoints as the core of occupational adaptation. Several occupational therapy theories described the value of adaptation as an inherent human process (Occupational Adaptation model; Schkade & Schultz, 1992), as a mechanism to achieve identity and competence (Model of Human Occupation; Kielhofner, 2008), as a means of making sense of the environment (Model of Sensory Processing; Dunn, 2007), and as a means of transacting with the environment (Ecology of Human Performance; Dunn, Brown & McGuigan, 1994). However, despite the rich body of literature describing adaptation as a universal construct in occupational therapy, there remain some challenges in the consistency of articulating, measuring, and using the construct in daily practice. This is why we conceptualized and developed this text.

In this book, we aim to present a multidimensional perspective to the construct of adaptation through occupation. In the different chapters, we use *occupational adaptation* to label this construct. We also seek to collectively assemble historical and contemporary occupational therapy, occupational science, and scientific research from neuroscience and other disciplines to demonstrate the potency of the process of adaptation through occupation. The book is arranged in four sections with 10 total chapters, methodically presenting an evolution of the construct. These sections are not meant to be timelines and do not necessarily present a chronological narrative of presenting information and discussions, but rather as organizers to help the reader approach knowledge and understanding of the construct based on carefully chosen themes. We do not expect that readers will consume information from the book methodically from one section and one chapter to another. Each chapter highlights a particular individual perspective with discussion points that may complement or critique other perspectives. As editors of the text, we preserved rather than minimized the varying and sometimes bold perspectives of the contributing authors to truly present the multidimensionality of the construct.

Section I presents a proposed dual perspective in defining occupational adaptation: a process that results in the transaction with the environment, and a measure of occupational participation. Section II aims to reframe existing neuroscience evidence on human adaptation as a result of goal-directed behaviors, task performance, repetitive activity, and meaningful engagement in occupations. This section also aims to justify that there is neural evidence to support the notion of occupational adaptation.

Section III presents four occupational therapy theories and models from a perspective of adaptation: Occupational Adaptation (OA; Chapter 5), Model of Human Occupation (MOHO; Chapter 6), Sensory Processing Model (Chapter 7), and Ecology of Human Performance (EHP; Chapter 8). We find that this section differs from any of the existing published occupational therapy theory books because of the emphasis and applied approach to understanding occupational adaptation. These theories and conceptual models were not chosen randomly to be part of this text; rather, they were selected because of their explicit discussions and perspectives on the adaptation process.

We like to think that Section IV brings heart to the book. This section provides an analysis of occupational science literature supporting adaptation while also using a series of research case studies to illustrate and exemplify the different definitions of occupational adaptation presented in this book. We wrote section overviews preceding the chapters so that each section is expanded further and the relationship of each chapter with the others is explained in further detail.

You may ask how one should make use of the contents of this book. We suggest different ways, and we challenge you to develop action steps! First, we hope that this book will help you become comfortable using the language of occupational adaptation or adaptation through occupation in your research, teaching, or practice. Each chapter begins with a proposed framing of occupational adaptation and a set of reflection and discussion questions to help frame applications of the chapter to daily practice. We hope that you are able to explain that many of the things we do in our daily occupational therapy practice is aimed not only at restoring or facilitating our clients' return to or achievement of function and participation in occupations, but also at enabling them to become more adaptive in life. With the changing landscape of health care reimbursement and shift from fee-based to value-based services, occupational therapists are in a unique position to improve quality and effective care by partnering with our clients to become more adaptive to independently solve challenges in daily life outside of the health care system. We hope that you are able to articulate ways to best measure the impact of occupational therapy on our clients' occupational adaptation. This might be through thoughtful use of assessment tools and development of clients' occupational profiles, development of new assessment tools, or careful documentation and articulation of changes in the adaptive functioning of our clients.

Second, we hope that educators using this book will find it beneficial in the teaching of occupational therapy and occupational science. We have provided PowerPoint presentation slides online that outline the contents of each of the chapters. These resources can be helpful for teaching content from this text.

We hope that when you teach occupational therapy theories, you will also highlight the construct of occupational adaptation embedded in several of them. We hope that when you teach human anatomy and neuroscience, you teach not only structures and implications to occupational performance, but also the implications on the adaptation process. We hope that when you teach concepts on occupation in introductory courses or occupational science courses, you will be able to share the rich body of knowledge about the construct.

Finally, if you are a researcher, scholar, or scientist, we hope that this book inspires critical thinking, discourse, and even debate on the ideas presented in this text. We encourage you to challenge, critique, and/or build on paradigms presented in this text, identify more gaps and help fill in these gaps, and contribute to increasing the body of knowledge on the construct of occupational adaptation.

Lenin C. Grajo, PhD, EdM, OTR/L
Angela K. Boisselle, PhD, OTR, ATP

REFERENCES

American Occupational Therapy Association. (2017). Philosophical base of occupational therapy. *American Journal of Occupational Therapy, 71*(Suppl. 2), 7112410045.

Dunn, W. (2007). *Living sensationally: Understanding your senses*. London, England: Jessica Kingsley Publishers.

Dunn, W., Brown, C., & McGuigan, A. (1994). The ecology of human performance: A framework for considering the effect of context. *American Journal of Occupational Therapy, 48*(7), 595-607.

Kielhofner, G. (2008). *Model of human occupation: Theory and application* (4th ed.). Philadelphia, PA: Lippincott Williams & Wilkins.

Schkade, J. K., & Schultz, S. (1992). Occupational adaptation: Toward a holistic approach for contemporary practice, part 1. *American Journal of Occupational Therapy, 46*(9), 829-837. doi:10.5014/ajot.46.9.829

Schultz, S., & Schkade, J. (1997). Adaptation. In C. Christiansen & C. Baum (Eds.), *Occupational therapy: Enabling function and well-being* (2nd ed., pp. 458-481). Thorofare, NJ: SLACK Incorporated.

Meyer, A. (1977). The philosophy of occupation therapy. *American Journal of Occupational Therapy, 31*(10), 639-642. (Reprinted from Archives of Occupational Therapy, 1922, 1, pp. 1-10.)

Yerxa, E. J. (1992). Some implications of occupational therapy's history for its epistemology, values and relation to medicine. *American Journal of Occupational Therapy, 46*(1), 79-83.

Section I

CONCEPTUAL EVOLUTION OF OCCUPATIONAL ADAPTATION

Angela K. Boisselle, PhD, OTR, ATP and Lenin C. Grajo, PhD, EdM, OTR/L

OVERVIEW

The first section will explore prominent occupational therapy and occupational science literature on the construct of occupational adaptation and methods of assessment used to measure the construct. Chapter 1 emphasizes the conceptual evolution of the construct of occupational adaptation from the beginning of the occupational therapy profession to the present day. This chapter was originally published as Grajo, Boisselle, and DaLomba's (2018) scoping study in the *Open Journal of Occupational Therapy*. The chapter introduces the purpose of this book through grounding definitions of adaptation and the themes prominent in literature. The chapter will set the groundwork for Chapter 2 through an introduction of various research methods that propose how occupational adaptation can be measured in practice, education, and research.

Chapter 2 expands upon the literature highlighted in Chapter 1, with a focus on the manner in which adaptation is assessed in occupational therapy literature. Adaptation as an outcome of occupational therapy intervention will be highlighted through historical literature, review of qualitative and quantitative assessments tools that have been created, and clinical and observational studies. Several themes such as relative mastery, occupational identity and competence, and adaptive capacity are introduced in both chapters and continue to develop throughout the book.

1

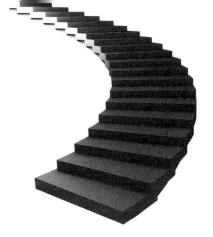

Defining the Construct of Occupational Adaptation

Lenin C. Grajo, PhD, EdM, OTR/L; Angela K. Boisselle, PhD, OTR, ATP; and Elaina DaLomba, PhD, MSW, OTR/L

OVERVIEW In this chapter, we synthesize as an introductory chapter the results of a scoping study on the construct of occupational adaptation that we published as an original research article in the *Open Journal of Occupational Therapy* (Grajo, Boisselle, & DaLomba, 2018). The study highlighted four essential definitions of the construct of occupational adaptation based on an analysis of 74 articles published in peer-reviewed publications. Occupational adaptation is defined as:

1. A product of engagement in occupation,
2. A transaction with the environment,
3. A manner of responding to change and life transitions,
4. And a process of forming a desired sense of self.

This chapter aims to provide an overview and synthesis, through a scoping study perspective, of the many expansions on the construct of occupational adaptation that you will read about throughout this text.

Grajo LC, Boisselle AK, eds.
Adaptation Through Occupation:
Multidimensional Perspectives (pp 3-18).
© 2019 SLACK Incorporated.

CHAPTER OBJECTIVES By the end of this chapter, the reader will be able to:
* Define occupational adaptation as a construct.
* Describe clinical and scholarly applications of the construct of occupational adaptation.
* Identify gaps in evidence and research about occupational adaptation.
* Identify ways by which educators, scholars, and clinicians can advance the knowledge and use of the construct of occupational adaptation.

QUESTIONS FOR DISCUSSION AND REFLECTION As the reader explores this chapter, let the following questions guide discussion and reflection:
* How do I define the construct of occupational adaptation and apply it in practice, teaching, and/or research?
* What are some challenges in understanding and applying the construct of occupational adaptation in practice, teaching, and/or research?

The contents of this chapter have been published in the *Open Journal of Occupational Therapy* as Grajo, L., Boisselle, A., & DaLomba, E. (2018). Occupational adaptation as a construct: A scoping review of literature. *Open Journal of Occupational Therapy, 6*(1). doi:10.15453/2168-6408.1400

DEFINING ADAPTATION

Adaptation is a critical construct in occupational therapy and occupational science. Definitions of adaptation in occupational therapy and occupational science literature have been varied and at times ambiguous. Occupational therapists often witness a transformative and personal process that occurs within the client when faced with diversity and change. Adaptation in this context is frequently used to define the internal human process as referenced in seminal literature. Meyer (1922/1977) asserted that many diseases of the 20th century are a result of problems of adaptation and that *meaningful work* can serve as "sovereign help" in helping patients become more adaptive (p. 639). Kielhofner (1980) described adaptation as an acquisition of competence. It is also viewed as a response to time and physical change (Fine, 1991; King, 1978); a source of meaning and motivation (Fine, 1991; Schultz & Schkade, 1997); and dependent upon the demands of the environment (Kielhofner, 2008; Schkade & Schultz, 1992). Adaptation has also been described in the literature as a method of modifying activities or tasks, making changes to the environment, and identifying the need for assistive equipment (Schultz & Schkade, 1997). However, this definition largely involves external influences on human occupation and not an internal human process that occurs during occupational participation.

Adaptation as a biological, sociological, and anthropological process has been well defined in the literature. The focus of this chapter, however, is to explore adaptation as a transformative process, internal to the person while participating in occupation and as an outcome of participation in occupation. As such, we will use the term *occupational adaptation* in this study to represent the construct as it relates to occupational participation.

OCCUPATIONAL ADAPTATION AS A PROCESS AND OUTCOME

Occupational Adaptation as a Process

Attempts to formalize occupational adaptation in terms of an internal process developed as part of occupational therapy theories as a means to understand humans as occupational beings. Two such theories are the Model of Human Occupation (MOHO) and Occupational Adaptation (OA) (see Chapters 5 and 6 for a full exploration of the construct based on these occupational therapy theories).

Kielhofner (1980) identified adaptation in MOHO as a construct that is temporal in nature that exists not only in childhood but also over a person's lifetime. Kielhofner also emphasized that identity and competence are established through interaction with the environment and are crucial to the adaptation process (2008). Kielhofner advocated that problems with adaptation, such as disability, require a readjustment of the person's identity and levels of competency.

Schkade and Schultz's OA model (1992) formally used the term *occupational adaptation* to define an internal and normative process and occupation as the means for adaptation. According to the model, human development involves a "continuous process of adaptation" based on the response to various occupational challenges (Schultz & Schkade, 1992, p. 918). Both MOHO and OA articulated that internal motivation and interaction with the environment help promote occupational adaptation. Authors from the academic discipline of occupational science echoed these principles but further connected the impact of occupational adaptation on participation and health (see Chapters 9 and 10 for occupational science perspectives on the construct).

In occupational science literature, Frank (1996) conceived that adaptation through occupation is fundamental to occupational science. She stated that as an internal process, when an individual encounters environmental challenges, the individual forms a series of adaptive responses. Frank proposed a definition of adaptation for occupational science that bridges the importance of occupational participation to impact health and well-being: "Adaptation is a process of selecting or organizing occupations to improve life opportunities and enhance quality of life" (p. 50).

Occupational Adaptation as an Outcome of Occupational Participation

Building on Frank's (1996) definition of adaptation, Wilcock's (1998) powerful work, "Reflections on Doing, Being and Becoming," seemed to propose adaptation as an outcome of occupational participation. Wilcock advocated for an expanded view of *becoming* within the practice of occupational therapy as a transformative process for human potential. Humans experience "becoming through doing and being" (p. 155). Adaptation is characterized as the change agent for the person and becomes an outcome of active engagement in occupation in pursuit of health.

Schkade and Schultz (1992) also articulated that the role of the occupational therapist is to empower the person to develop his or her own sense of relative mastery in order to transact with the environment. *Relative mastery* is the manner in which the person utilizes time and energy (efficiency), produces desired results (effectiveness), and achieves internal and external satisfaction during occupational performance (Schultz & Schkade, 1997). The authors described that relative mastery and increased adaptive capacity are outcomes of effective occupational therapy intervention. According to the model, increased adaptiveness should be the outcome of occupational therapy programming (Schkade & Schultz, 2003).

Similar to Wilcock (1998) and Schkade and Schultz (1992), Nelson (1997) articulated that occupational engagement has the power to alter a person's being, and the occupational therapist has a critical role in the adaptive process by providing optimal opportunities for engagement. Although the occupational therapist acts to facilitate adaptation, it is ultimately the client's self-initiated process of engagement through occupation that results in adaptation (Frank, 1996; Nelson, 1997). With this in mind, it is reasonable that occupational adaptation be used to promote positive change and health within the client, an *outcome* of the process.

The construct of occupational adaptation appears to be important in the history, body of knowledge, and identity building of occupational therapy and occupational science. What is not clear is whether those beliefs are still relevant and, if so, how those beliefs are translated—applied and understood—into practice.

Is Occupational Adaptation Still Used in Practice?

Shannon (1977) cautions us against the *derailment* of our profession by minimizing the influence of adaptation. He called for a recommitment to our foundational values and beliefs. King (1978) also proclaimed that adaptation is a fundamental concept in occupational therapy and called for the rigorous analysis of adaptation through research. Despite the historical underpinnings of occupational adaptation within our profession, recent literature and documents from the American Occupational Therapy Association (AOTA) provide scant reference to the construct. AOTA's revised statement of the philosophical base of occupational therapy (2011) and Distinct Value Statement (2015) refer to engagement and participation in occupation but stop short of mentioning occupational adaptation as an important process of occupational participation. The third edition of the Occupational Therapy Practice Framework (OTPF-III) refers to adaptation in a simplified manner of modification of the task or environment (AOTA, 2014). Only in the latest revision of the Philosophical Base of Occupational Therapy (AOTA, 2017) has adaptation been described as an outcome of occupational participation.

In a reconceptualization of the Schkade and Schultz OA model, Grajo (2017) asserted that the reason the model and construct seemed to be difficult to translate into practice is the complex terminologies used to describe occupational adaptation as a process. Grajo proposed that the principles of the model be simplified and better described as a feature of normative human development (an internal process) and as a way to describe the result of occupational therapy intervention (outcome). For more details about Schkade and Schultz's model, see Chapter 5 of this text.

The primary motivation of our research is to examine several questions on the use of the construct of occupational adaptation through a scoping review of literature. Some questions that guided our framing of this study and the development of our primary research questions include the following:

- Is occupational adaptation still a relevant construct in understanding human occupation?
- Is the redirection away from the use of the construct due to difficulty in translating it from theory into practice?
- Is the lack of a uniform definition of occupational adaptation hindering its articulation in practice?
- Is there evidence that we can use occupational adaptation not only as a process but as an outcome of therapy?
- Are we currently applying rigorous research on this construct?

In this scoping study, we aim to present implications on how occupational adaptation can be applied more effectively in clinical practice.

THE SCOPING STUDY ON OCCUPATIONAL ADAPTATION

In the following section, we report findings based on a scoping study we conducted to explore existing literature on occupational adaptation. Figure 1-1 shows the database search process and selection criteria for reviews of selected articles. We chose a scoping study research design to allow us to examine the extent, range, and nature of research activity and identify gaps in the literature (Arksey & O'Malley, 2005) on the construct of occupational adaptation. We believe that there is a rich body of literature in occupational therapy and occupational science exploring definitions and clinical applications of occupational adaptation, but this literature has yet to be synthesized and reviewed. We used Arksey and O'Malley's five-stage scoping study framework (2005) in our research process: (1) identifying the research questions; (2) identifying relevant studies; (3) selecting studies; (4) charting the data; and (5) collating, summarizing, and reporting results. For a full description of the methodologies for the scoping study, we invite the reader to refer to the published study in the *Open Journal of Occupational Therapy*.

Research Questions

- How is the construct of occupational adaptation defined and applied in different areas of occupational therapy practice?
- What are potential gaps in the literature on the application and use of occupational adaptation as a construct in the literature?

Figure 1-1. Scoping study search strategy and selection process for the reviews.

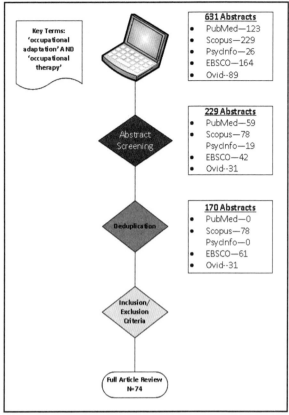

Applications of Occupational Adaptation in the Literature: Scoping Study Results

To respond to our research question on how the construct of occupational adaptation is defined and applied in different areas of occupational therapy practice, we present quantitative results in three subsections: (1) study designs used, (2) relevant literature influences, and (3) applications of occupational adaptation based on our *a-priori* definitions of process and outcome. Table 1-1 provides a summary of frequency tallies of all studies based on the aforementioned criteria.

Study Designs

For the first analysis, we examined the type of study design for each article. More than half of the studies analyzed were qualitative/descriptive in nature (n = 40). None were randomized, controlled trials. Two studies were systematic literature reviews.

Table 1-1

Frequency Analysis of Occupational Adaptation Studies	
Scoping Study Analysis Criteria	**(n)**
Study design	Mixed methods (13)
	Qualitative/descriptive (40)
	Case studies and single subject (7)
	Group, nonrandomized (5)
	Group, randomized (0)
	Lit reviews, scoping/systematic reviews (9)
Relevant literature influences[a]	Fidler & Fidler, 1978 (2)
	Frank, 1996 (6)
	Kielhofner, 1995, 2002, 2008 (17)
	Kielhofner & Burke, 1980 (2)
	Kielhofner, 1977 (2)
	Kielhofner, 1992, 1997, 2004 (4)
	Kielhofner, 1995 (2)
	King, 1978 (3)
	Meyer, 1922/1977 (4)
	Nelson, 1988 (5)
	Nelson, 1996 (2)
	Nelson, 1997 (3)
	Reed, 1984 (2)
	Reilly, 1962 (2)
	Rogers, 1983 (2)
	Schkade & McClung, 2001 (8)
	Schkade & Schultz, 1992 (41)
	Schultz & Schkade, 1992 (18)
	Schultz & Schkade, 1997 (7)
	Wilcock, 1998, 2006 (5)
	Wood, 1996 (3)
Use of occupational adaptation as a construct	Internal process (49)
	Outcome (37)
	Both internal process and outcome (12)
	Other (not clearly defined) (4)
Study participants	With medical conditions (788)
	Without medical conditions (904)
	Health care workers, educators (72)
	Instrument development (389)

[a]Full list of relevant literature can be found in Grajo, L., Boisselle, A., & DaLomba, E. (2018). Occupational adaptation as a construct: A scoping review of literature. *Open Journal of Occupational Therapy*, 6(1). doi:10.15453/2168-6408.1400

Relevant Literature Citations and Definitions of Occupational Adaptation

Publications related to the OA model (Schkade & Schultz, 1992) were the most commonly cited literature to define occupational adaptation (74 times from four different publications). Frequently cited constructs from the OA model from the 74 citations included adaptive strategies, press for mastery, and occupational adaptation as an internal normative process. MOHO (Kielhofner, 2008) publications were cited 27 times in various studies. Identity and competence were commonly cited constructs from the 27 studies. Other regularly cited literature from the studies in the scoping review included occupational science perspectives (Frank, 1996; Wilcock, 2006) and Nelson's perspectives on occupational identity and meaning (1997).

Applications and Definitions of Occupational Adaptation in Occupational Therapy Practice

Of the 74 studies reviewed, 49 used occupational adaptation to describe the internal process that occurs during participation in occupations. Thirty-seven studies described occupational adaptation as an outcome or result of increased or renewed participation in occupations. Twelve studies described occupational adaptation as both a process and outcome. Four studies briefly alluded to occupational adaptation as an internal process related to occupational therapy clinical reasoning or process during adaptation of the environment.

The lived experience of the process of occupational adaptation during participation in occupations (61%, n = 45) was a common theme found in the scoping review. These studies included participants with existing medical conditions (n = 788 aggregated from all 74 studies) and those without medical conditions (e.g., migrants, incarcerated populations; n = 904 aggregated from all 74 studies). Twelve studies looked at the impact of various occupational therapy interventions in the occupational adaptation of participants. Of the studies reviewed, only five were related to the development of occupational therapy instruments.

DEFINING OCCUPATIONAL ADAPTATION: THEMES FROM THE LITERATURE

This qualitative section aims to present analysis to respond to our first research question identifying how occupational adaptation is defined and applied in literature and to aid in responding to the research question on identifying the gaps in literature. Four themes emerged from the thematic analysis of codes from all 74 studies offering definitions of occupational adaptation as a process and outcome: (1) a product of engagement in occupations, (2) a process that emerges during transaction with the environment, (3) a manner of responding to change and life transitions, and (4) a process to form a desired sense of self. Because of the volume of studies in the scoping review, we chose to only cite a few exemplary studies to justify the common themes from all studies.

Theme 1: A Product of Engagement, Finding Meaning and Satisfaction in Occupations

Occupational adaptation was defined in the literature as a process of selecting and organizing activities (Lentin, 2006), a process of altering the meaning of engagement and changing the occupation itself (Beagan & Hattie, 2015; Norberg, Boman, Löfgren, & Brännström, 2014), and a construct to define occupation as meaningful and requiring active participation from the person (Dolecheck & Schkade, 1999; Hoogerdijk, Runge, & Haugboelle, 2011). Participants in various studies experienced the process of occupational adaptation through the need to re-engage and redefine the meaning of important occupations during transitional periods in life such as coming out as a lesbian, gay, bisexual, or transgender (Beagan & Hattie, 2015) or following a stroke (Dolecheck & Schkade, 1999) or congestive heart failure (Norberg et al., 2014).

Theme 2: Emerges From the Transaction With the Environment

Occupational adaptation was identified as a mechanism to manage and respond to the occupational environment (Brayman, 1996; Spencer, Davidson, & White, 1996) and a manner of receiving validation from the environment (Taylor et al., 2003). From a therapeutic perspective, occupational adaptation was applied and defined as the process of adapting the self and the environment to provide holistic care or intervention (Dale et al., 2002). Crist et al. (2005) reinforced the environment as a significant influence on the occupational adaptation process. Using perspectives from individuals who have experienced various life-altering situations, Spencer, Davidson, and White (1996) defined occupational adaptation as knowing how to respond to different challenges based on familiarity of the environment. The authors also expanded on how occupational adaptation forms *occupational repertoire*—or sets of forms that create memories—and *cumulative repertoire*—or memories that change one's sense of competence and mastery—as a result of building a relationship with the occupational environment. In a study of adults with chronic fatigue syndrome, Taylor et al. (2003) also explored the manner in which participants navigated through adaptive transitions. As a result, adaptation transpires through the presence of social support and validation from environment.

Instrument development studies that measure occupational adaptation also supported the importance of the occupational adaptation process. In developing the Relative Mastery Measurement Scale, George, Schkade, and Ishee (2004) emphasized the use of self-selected activities to increase engagement and increased awareness of new or modified responses to environmental demands as key features of the occupational adaptation process. In developing the Occupational Performance History Interview, Mallinson, Mahaffey, and Kielhofner (1998) also found the influence of the environment to be strong enough to warrant its assessment as a unique construct of the occupational adaptation process.

Theme 3: A Manner of Responding to Change, Altered Situations, Life Transitions

Occupational adaptation was described in a majority of the studies as a manner of coping and being resilient and as a use of appropriate strategies in response to altered or changing life situations (Dale et al., 2002; Nayar & Stanley, 2015). Several authors framed occupational adaptation during the presence of adverse life events as a result of engagement in occupations necessary for healing (Ammann, Satink, & Andresen, 2012); a manner of reestablishing life balance (Gruwsved, Söderback, & Fernholm, 1996); a process of overcoming disabling influences on occupational functioning (Bontje, Kinebanian, Josephsson, & Tamura, 2004); an iterative process of occupational accommodation and occupational assimilation as experienced in a sense of loss (Hoppes & Segal, 2010); and a process of reclaiming roles and participating in alternate occupations (Gibbs, Boshoff, & Stanley, 2015). In a grounded theory study approach to understand the experiences of immigrant women, Nayar and Stanley (2015) defined occupational adaptation as a strategy to proactively respond to altered situations and broaden one's occupational choices. The authors focused on occupational adaptation as a social process related to redefining self-identity during a period of change rather than a state of functioning (see Chapter 10). Ammann et al. (2012) narrated how adults with significant hand injuries individually "recaptured" occupational life at their own pace, striving for normality as fast as possible, and offered occupational adaptation as multiple redefinitions of self and abilities needed throughout process of healing. A study of adults with different physical disabilities by Bontje et al. (2004) defined occupational adaptation as a process of overcoming disabling influences on occupational functioning. Their findings contrast the theoretical discourse on occupational adaptation focused on the personal adaptiveness, suggesting that occupational adaptation is a two-fold process in which the social environment also adapts to reduce effects of disabling influences on person's occupational function. Hoppes and Segal (2010) found that individuals reconstruct meaning in occupations following loss in order to maintain well-being. Gibbs et al. (2015) asserted that it is through participation in occupation that people generate and express visions of possibility to resolve occupational challenges, and this process leads to occupational adaptation.

Theme 4: Formation of Desired Sense of Self, Competence, Mastery, and Identity

Occupational adaptation was defined in the literature as an ongoing, nonlinear process to achieve a desired sense of self (Lexell, Iwarsson, & Lund, 2011); a manner of developing a sense of competence, self-efficacy, and identity within occupational participation (Crist et al., 2005; Firfirey & Hess-April, 2014; Johansson & Isaksson, 2011; Yazdani, 2011); and a manner of reframing identity, competence, the environment, and the fit between all three (Klinger, 2005; Mallinson et al., 1998). Additionally, Luck and Beagan (2015) asserted the reciprocal process between occupational adaptation and identity. In a study of adults who experienced long-term hospitalization due to tuberculosis, Firfirey and Hess-April (2014) explored the narratives of the participants, the process of occupational adaptation, and how it impacted their sense of identity. The hospitalization brought about a sense of loss due to many unmet occupational needs and the lack of occupational choices to fulfill many important life roles. The study also exemplified how disability facilitates the need to overcome barriers to occupational adaptation using various personal factors such as resilience and spirituality. Klinger (2005) defined occupational adaptation as the process of change—the process of "I am not who I was before" to becoming "I have to accept the new me"—as a result of traumatic brain injury. Klinger's study also explored how this shift in identity caused by disability facilitated the "change in the ways of doing" occupations of the participants (2005).

WHAT DOES THE BODY OF KNOWLEDGE TELL US ABOUT OUR UNDERSTANDING OF OCCUPATIONAL ADAPTATION?

The quantitative findings in our study indicate a rich body of relevant literature that offer various definitions and applications of occupational adaptation as a construct. The application of occupational adaptation has been seen to not only understand the process of illness, disease, or disability in populations with medical conditions. The construct has also been widely used to understand the normative process of occupational adaptation in different populations without medical conditions.

Our qualitative findings suggest that defining occupational adaptation as a process and outcome is complex, and the constructs are difficult to dichotomize in terms of these definitions. These confounding issues have perhaps contributed to the profession's deviation away from the construct in more recent years. Studies describing the lived experience of occupational adaptation identified the construct as both a product (outcome) of engagement in occupations and the ability to find meaning and satisfaction in those (process). Moreover, occupational adaptation emerges from interactions within the environment (both a process and outcome) and in response to evolving environmental demands, which impact occupational status. These themes deeply resonated with Schkade and Schultz's (1992), Frank's (1996), and Nelson's (1997) perspectives on the occupational adaptation process. The transcendent process of engagement, re-engagement, or altered engagement to fulfill a desire to reestablish identity, competence, and mastery over situations and occupations were consistent throughout the studies. This indicates that occupational adaptation can both be an internal process and an outcome of occupational participation. These assertions are also echoed in the perspectives of Kielhofner (2008), Meyer (1922/1977), and Wilcock (1998).

Our scoping review found three gaps in the literature. First, there is a lack of clarity in articulating how occupational adaptation is defined and used in many of the studies in this scoping review. Although there is a common theme defining occupational adaptation as an important construct in occupational participation, several studies do not explicitly frame the construct as a process within a person that allows him or her to respond to the different challenges of occupational participation or the outcome—an increase in adaptive capacity—as a result of the challenges in occupational participation.

This lack of clarity resonates in the assertion by Grajo (2017) in his reconceptualization of the Schkade and Schultz (1992) model that without specificity when defining the construct as a process, an outcome, or a process and outcome of occupational participation or occupational therapy intervention, occupational adaptation will remain a construct that is difficult to "name and frame" in daily clinical practice. This naming and framing challenge may be the reason for the next two gaps we found in the literature.

The second gap is a significant lack of studies measuring the impact of intervention in clients' occupational adaptation. Although limited in number, the outcome measurement studies in our scoping review support the thematic findings defining the construct as an outcome of intervention, and the majority of these included analysis of the lived experience of occupational adaptation in clinical and nonclinical applications. Several intervention studies for medical conditions (e.g., cerebrovascular accident, multiple sclerosis, and chronic pain) noted functional gains (outcome) as well changes in mindfulness and perceived well-being (process). The qualitative data from these articles further support the nonindependent and nonexclusive nature of the two (process and outcome) as we have discussed earlier. This idea is highly consistent with the original principles of Schkade and Schultz's OA model (1992).

The third gap is the lack of published and developed instruments to measure occupational adaptation. The lack of published assessments may be a result of the complexity and vague definitions of the construct. However, the few published instrument development studies add support to the importance of the process. For example, in the Relative Mastery Measurement Scale based on the OA model (George et al., 2004), occupational adaptation was viewed as a normative process that develops and changes as individuals seek relative mastery. Occupational adaptation was viewed as a process that leads to occupational identity and competence in the MOHO and was a guiding construct in the development of the Occupational Circumstances Assessment Interview and Rating Scale (Lai, Haglund, & Kielhofner, 1999) and the revision of the Occupational Performance History Interview (Mallinson et al., 1998). The goal of the aforementioned tools, directly and indirectly, is to measure the temporal progression of the individual's occupational adaptation during participation in occupations.

LIMITATIONS

The primary limitation of this study was the subtle differences in the way in which occupational therapists define and use the terms *occupation*, *adaptation*, and *occupational adaptation* that made the literature search and analysis complex. The authors constantly brainstormed and discussed how to differentiate the construct as an outcome or process when used in the studies. These subjective discussions may have inherent biases that influenced the way we thematically analyzed and coded the studies. We also searched only five databases (after finding redundancy in many of them). Searches with other terms and other databases may have yielded more or different sets of articles for review.

ADVANCING THE KNOWLEDGE ON OCCUPATIONAL ADAPTATION

Occupational adaptation is applied in contemporary literature to understand the transactional process between the person, occupations, and environment and an outcome of occupational participation. Occupational adaptation is a complex and abstract construct, and this can make researching the construct challenging. However, occupational adaptation remains central to the identity of the profession. It is imperative to examine how it is operationalized and evaluated in the therapeutic process and articulated in the essential roles of occupational therapy to its stakeholders to continue developing the body of knowledge on occupational adaptation and to highlight how occupational adaptation is a defining construct in articulating the distinct value of occupational therapy.

Occupational adaptation is a historically rooted and important construct in occupational therapy literature. However, there is a lack of clarity in the use and definition of the construct of occupational adaptation. This construct can be better articulated in the philosophical base of occupational therapy and when publishing studies that describe and measure the construct.

SUMMARY AND IMPLICATIONS

- Occupational adaptation is an important construct that needs to be routinely and clearly articulated as a process and outcome of treatment based on occupational participation: Occupational adaptation is a process. The process of occupational adaptation allows us to navigate challenges of daily occupational performance and transact with the occupational environment. Occupational adaptation is an outcome of occupational participation. Occupational adaptation creates a desired sense of self and a sense of competence and mastery and this construct can be used to further support the profession's distinct value of improving health and quality of life.

- Facilitation of occupational participation and engagement are not the only means to improve health and well-being. Occupational therapists need to enable the adaptiveness of their clients as well. This process needs to be more clearly described in research studies. Clients who are adaptive are able to choose and engage in occupations that are meaningful to them, respond to life's challenges and adversities, and navigate their environment with mastery. These markers are outcomes of occupational therapy intervention and can be used as means to describe occupational adaptation as an outcome.

- Our study found that there are significant gaps in the literature in the area of outcomes research that demonstrate how occupational therapists facilitate occupational adaptation. Further research is needed to define occupational therapy's unique role in maintaining and promoting health and the occupational adaptation of clients. Research on intervention effectiveness and outcomes of intervention on occupational adaptiveness can further strengthen the growing body of evidence on this construct.

- When occupational adaptation is clearly articulated and defined in research, the construct can be more clearly measured and more instruments can be developed. Because occupational therapy is an evidenced-based profession, occupational therapists need to use the tools available to assess the outcomes of occupational therapy intervention on the occupational adaptation process of clients. More valid and reliable tools that can measure the multiple facets of occupational adaptation such as occupational competence and identity (MOHO) and relative mastery (OA model) in relation to occupational adaptation are needed.

REFERENCES

American Occupational Therapy Association. (2011). The philosophical base of occupational therapy. *American Journal of Occupational Therapy, 65*(Suppl.), S65. doi:10.5014/ajot.2011.65S65

American Occupational Therapy Association. (2014). Occupational therapy practice framework: Domain and process (3rd ed.). *American Journal of Occupational Therapy, 68*(Suppl. 1), S1-S48. doi:10.5014/ajot.2014.682006

American Occupational Therapy Association. (2015). Articulating the distinct value of occupational therapy. Retrieved from https://www.aota.org/Publications-News/AOTANews/2015/distinct-value-of-occupational-therapy.aspx

American Occupational Therapy Association. (2017). Philosophical base of occupational therapy. *American Journal of Occupational Therapy, 71*(Suppl. 2), 7112410045. doi:10.5014/ajot.2017.716S06

Ammann, B., Satink, T., & Andresen, M. (2012). Experiencing occupations with chronic hand disability: Narratives of hand-injured adults. *Hand Therapy, 17*(4), 87-94. doi:10.1177/1758998312471253

Arksey, H., & O'Malley, L. (2005). Scoping studies: Towards a methodological framework. *International Journal of Social Research Methodology, 8*(1), 19-32. doi:10.1080/1364557032000119616

Beagan, B. L., & Hattie, B. (2015). LGBTQ experiences with religion and spirituality: Occupational transition and adaptation. *Journal of Occupational Science, 22*(4), 459-476. doi:10.1080/14427591.2014.953670

Bontje, P., Kinebanian, A., Josephsson, S., & Tamura, Y. (2004). Occupational adaptation: The experiences of older persons with physical disabilities. *American Journal of Occupational Therapy, 58*(2), 140-149. doi:10.5014/ajot.58.2.140

Brayman, S. J. (1996). Managing the occupational environment of managed care. *American Journal of Occupational Therapy, 50*(6), 442-446. doi:10.5014/ajot.50.6.442

Crist, P., Fairman, A., Muñoz, J. P., Witchger Hansen, A. M., Sciulli, J., & Eggers, M. (2005). Education and practice collaborations: A pilot case study between a university faculty and county jail practitioners. *Occupational Therapy in Health Care, 19*(1-2), 193-210. doi:10.1080/J003v19n01_14

Dale, L. M., Fabrizio, A. J., Adhlakha, P., Mahon, M. K., McGraw, E. E., Neyenhaus, R. D., … Zaber, J. M. (2002). Occupational therapists working in hand therapy: The practice of holism in a cost containment environment. *Work, 19*(1), 35-45.

Dolecheck, J. R., & Schkade, J. K. (1999). The extent dynamic standing endurance is effected when CVA subjects perform personally meaningful activities rather than nonmeaningful tasks. *Occupational Therapy Journal of Research, 19*(1), 40-54.

Fidler, G. S., & Fidler, J. W. (1978). Doing and becoming: Purposeful action and self-actualization. *American Journal of Occupational Therapy, 32*(5), 305-310. doi:10.5014/ajot.64.1.142

Fine, S. B. (1991). Resilience and human adaptability: Who rises above adversity? *American Journal of Occupational Therapy, 45*(6), 493-503. doi:10.5014/ajot.45.6.493

Firfirey, N., & Hess-April, L. (2014). A study to explore the occupational adaptation of adults with MDR-TB who undergo long-term hospitalisation. *South African Journal of Occupational Therapy, 44*(3), 18-24.

Frank, G. (1996). The concept of adaptation as a foundation for occupational science. In R. Zemke & F. Clark (Eds.), *Occupational science: An evolving discipline* (pp. 47-55). Philadelphia, PA: F.A. Davis.

George, L. A., Schkade, J. K., & Ishee, J. H. (2004). Content validity of the relative mastery measurement scale: A measure of occupational adaptation. *Occupational Therapy Journal of Research*, *24*(3), 92-102.

Gibbs, D., Boshoff, K., & Stanley, M. (2015). Becoming the parent of a preterm infant: A meta-ethnographic synthesis. *British Journal of Occupational Therapy*, *78*(8), 475-487. doi:10.1177/0308022615586799

Grajo, L. (2017). Occupational adaptation. In J. Hinojosa, P. Kramer, & C. Royeen (Eds.), *Perspectives on human occupation: Theories underlying practice* (2nd ed., pp. 287-311). Philadelphia, PA: F.A. Davis.

Gruwsved, Å., Söderback, I., & Fernholm, C. (1996). Evaluation of a vocational training programme in primary health care rehabilitation: A case study. *Work*, *7*(1), 47-61.

Hoogerdijk, B., Runge, U., & Haugboelle, J. (2011). The adaptation process after traumatic brain injury an individual and ongoing occupational struggle to gain a new identity. *Scandinavian Journal of Occupational Therapy*, *18*(2), 122-132. doi:10.3109/11038121003645985

Hoppes, S., & Segal, R. (2010). Reconstructing meaning through occupation after the death of a family member: Accommodation, assimilation, and continuing bonds. *American Journal of Occupational Therapy*, *64*(1), 133-141. doi:10.5014/ajot.64.1.133

Johansson, C., & Isaksson, G. (2011). Experiences of participation in occupations of women on long-term sick leave. *Scandinavian Journal of Occupational Therapy*, *18*(4), 294-301. doi:10.3109/11038128.2010.521950

Kielhofner, G. (1977). Temporal adaptation: A conceptual framework for occupational therapy. *American Journal of Occupational Therapy*, *31*(4), 235-242.

Kielhofner, G. (1980). Model of human occupation, part 2. Ontogenesis from the perspective of temporal adaptation. *American Journal of Occupational Therapy*, *34*(10), 657-663. doi:10.5014/ajot.34.10.657

Kielhofner, G. (1992). *Conceptual foundations of occupational therapy*. Philadelphia, PA: F.A. Davis.

Kielhofner, G. (1995). *A model of human occupation: Theory and application* (2nd ed.). Baltimore, MD: Lippincott Williams & Wilkins.

Kielhofner, G (1997). *Conceptual foundations of occupational therapy* (2nd ed.). Philadelphia, PA: F.A. Davis.

Kielhofner, G. (2002). *A model of human occupation: Theory and application* (3rd ed.). Baltimore, MD: Lippincott Williams & Wilkins.

Kielhofner, G (2004). *Conceptual foundations of occupational therapy*. (3rd ed.). Philadelphia, PA: F.A. Davis.

Kielhofner, G. (2008). *A model of human occupation: Theory and application* (4th ed.). Philadelphia, PA: Lippincott Williams & Wilkins.

Kielhofner, G., & Burke, J. (1980). A model of human occupation, part 1. *American Journal of Occupational Therapy*, *34*(9), 572-581.

King, L. J. (1978). 1978 Eleanor Clarke Slagle Lecture: Toward a science of adaptive responses. *American Journal of Occupational Therapy*, *32*, 429-437.

Klinger, L. (2005). Occupational adaptation: Perspectives of people with traumatic brain injury. *Journal of Occupational Science*, *12*(1), 9-16.

Lai, J. S., Haglund, L., & Kielhofner, G. (1999). Occupational case analysis interview and rating scale: An examination of construct validity. *Scandinavian Journal of Caring Science*, *13*, 267-273.

Lentin, P. (2006). Occupational terminology. *Journal of Occupational Science*, *13*(2), 153-157. doi:10.1080/14427591.2005.9686564

Lexell, E. M., Iwarsson, S., & Lund, M. L. (2011). Occupational adaptation in people with multiple sclerosis. *OTJR: Occupation, Participation and Health*, *31*(3), 127-134. doi:10.3928/15394492-20101025-01

Luck, K., & Beagan, B. (2015). Occupational transition of smoking cessation in women: 'you're restructuring your whole life.' *Journal of Occupational Science*, *22*(2), 183-196. doi:10.1080/14427591.2014.887418

Mallinson, T., Mahaffey, L., & Kielhofner, G. (1998). The occupational performance history interview: Evidence for three underlying constructs of occupational adaptation. *Canadian Journal of Occupational Therapy*, *65*(4), 219-228. doi:10.1177/000841749806500407

Meyer, A. (1977). The philosophy of occupation therapy. *American Journal of Occupational Therapy*, *31*(10), 639-642. (Reprinted from Archives of Occupational Therapy, 1922, 1, pp. 1-10.)

Nayar, S., & Stanley, M. (2015). Occupational adaptation as a social process in everyday life. *Journal of Occupational Science*, *22*(1), 26-38. doi:10.1080/14427591.2014.882251

Nelson, D. L. (1988). Occupation: Form and performance. *American Journal of Occupational Therapy*, *42*, 633-641. doi:10.5014/ajot.42.10.633

Nelson, D. L. (1996). Therapeutic occupation: A definition. *American Journal of Occupational Therapy,* *50*(10), 775-782.

Nelson, D. L. (1997). Why the profession of occupational therapy will flourish in the 21st Century. The 1996 Eleanor Clark Slagle Lecture. *American Journal of Occupational Therapy, 51,* 11-24. doi:10.5014/ajot.51.1.11

Norberg, E., Boman, K., Löfgren, B., & Brännström, M. (2014). Occupational performance and strategies for managing daily life among the elderly with heart failure. *Scandinavian Journal of Occupational Therapy, 21*(5), 392-399. doi:10.3109/11038128.2014.911955

Reed, K. L. (1984). *Models of practice in occupational therapy.* Baltimore, MD: Lippincott Williams & Wilkins.

Reilly, M. (1962). Occupational therapy can be one of the great ideas of 20th century medicine. *American Journal of Occupational Therapy, 16,* 1-9.

Rogers, J. C. (1983). Eleanor Clarke Slagle Lectureship—1983; clinical reasoning: the ethics, science, and art. *American Journal of Occupational Therapy, 37*(9), 601-616.

Schkade, J., & McClung, M. (2001). *Occupational adaptation in practice: Concepts and cases.* Thorofare, NJ: SLACK Incorporated.

Schkade, J. K., & Schultz, S. (1992). Occupational adaptation: Toward a holistic approach for contemporary practice, part 1. *American Journal of Occupational Therapy, 46*(9), 829-837. doi:10.5014/ajot.46.9.829

Schkade, J. K., & Schultz, S. (2003). Occupational adaptation. In P. Kramer, J. Hinojosa, & C. B. Royeen (Eds.), *Perspectives in human occupation: Participation in life* (pp. 181-221). Baltimore, MD: Lippincott Williams & Wilkins.

Schultz, S., & Schkade, J. (1997). Adaptation. In C. Christiansen & C. Baum (Eds.), *Occupational therapy: Enabling function and well-being* (2nd ed., pp. 459-481). Thorofare, NJ: SLACK Incorporated.

Schultz, S., & Schkade, J. K. (1992). Occupational adaptation: Toward a holistic approach for contemporary practice, part 2. *American Journal of Occupational Therapy, 46*(10), 917-925. doi:10.5014/ajot.46.10.917

Shannon, P. D. (1977). The derailment of occupational therapy. *American Journal of Occupational Therapy, 31,* 229-234.

Spencer, J. C., Davidson, H. A., & White, V. K. (1996). Continuity and change: Past experience as adaptive repertoire in occupational adaptation. *American Journal of Occupational Therapy, 50*(7), 526-534. doi:10.5014/ajot.50.7.526

Taylor, R. R., Kielhofner, G. W., Abelenda, J., Colantuono, K., Fong, T., Heredia, R., … Vazquez, E. (2003). An approach to persons with chronic fatigue syndrome based on the model of human occupation: Part one, impact on occupational performance and participation. *Occupational Therapy in Health Care, 17*(2), 47-61. doi:10.1080/J003v17n02_04

Wilcock, A. (2006). *An occupational perspective of health* (2nd ed.). Thorofare, NJ: SLACK Incorporated.

Wilcock, A. A. (1998). Reflections on doing, being and becoming. *Canadian Journal of Occupational Therapy, 65*(5), 248-256. doi:10.1177/000841749806500501

Wood, W. (1996). Legitimizing occupational therapy's knowledge. *American Journal of Occupational Therapy, 50*(8), 626-634.

Yazdani, F. (2011). How students with low level subjective wellbeing perceive the impact of the environment on occupational behaviour. *International Journal of Therapy and Rehabilitation, 18*(8), 462-469. doi:10.12968/ijtr.2011.18.8.462

2

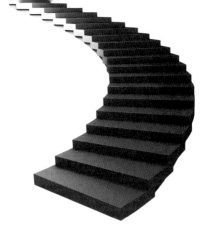

Adaptation as a Measure of Occupational Participation

Lorrie George-Paschal, PhD, OTR/L, ATP and
Lenin C. Grajo, PhD, EdM, OTR/L

OVERVIEW In this chapter, we analyze many of the studies included in the scoping review of literature presented in Chapter 1 and offer an analysis of occupational adaptation as an outcome of occupational participation. Occupational adaptation is a construct that can be measured using quantitative tools and qualitative methodologies. Three themes emerged from a review of evidence and research on how occupational adaptation is measured: (1) a measure of relative mastery, (2) a measure of occupational identity and competence, and (3) a measure of adaptive capacity.

CHAPTER OBJECTIVES By the end of this chapter, the reader will be able to:
- Articulate how occupational adaptation can be measured as an outcome of occupational participation.
- Define relative mastery as a measure of occupational adaptation.
- Define occupational identity and competence as measures of occupational
- adaptation.
- Define adaptive capacity as measure of occupational adaptation.

Grajo LC, Boisselle AK, eds.
Adaptation Through Occupation:
Multidimensional Perspectives (pp 19-31).
© 2019 SLACK Incorporated.

QUESTIONS FOR DISCUSSION AND REFLECTION As the reader explores this chapter, let the following questions guide discussion and reflection:
- Can occupational adaptation as a construct be measured?
- What assessments are currently available that measure occupational adaptation?
- Why do I need to measure the occupational adaptation of my clients?

INTRODUCTION

This chapter provides an overview of the assessment of the construct of occupational adaptation from a variety of perspectives. The scope of literature presented will traverse research traditions, theoretical boundaries, and operational definitions of the construct. Due to the critical role of measurement (Asher, 2014; Doucet & Gutman, 2013) for the survival of the profession, a discussion of key instruments that evaluate the construct is also included.

In this chapter, we offer different perspectives on how occupational adaptation can be measured using quantitative tools, descriptive tools, and qualitative methods. Outcomes-based and experimental research provide the scientific evidence needed to quantify results, whereas qualitative and descriptive methodologies increase our depth of understanding of the construct. Our knowledge of outcomes, combined with increased insight on the process of adaptation, may lead to best practice.

Three themes surrounding the assessment of occupational adaptation emerged from our analysis of the literature: (1) relative mastery, (2) occupational identity and occupational competence, and (3) adaptive capacity. Together these constructs provide a holistic view of man's adaptation leading to improved occupational functioning. The following review of the literature will discuss patterns of research within each of these themes, including relevant instruments designed to measure constructs.

RELATIVE MASTERY AS AN INDICATOR OF OCCUPATIONAL ADAPTATION

According to Schkade and Schultz's Occupational Adaptation (OA) model (Schkade & Schultz, 1992; Schultz, 2009), *relative mastery* and *adaptive capacity* are two primary indicators of improvement in occupational adaptation. Relative mastery is based on one's sense of *effectiveness, efficiency, and satisfaction to self and others*. A change in relative mastery is also said to be observable by others through signs of initiation in occupational performance and generalization of learned strategies in different contexts of occupation (Schultz & Schkade, 1992). Improved occupational adaptation is proposed to lead to increased occupational functioning (Schultz, 2014). As an outcome of intervention based on the OA model, relative mastery has been evaluated quantitatively and qualitatively with a variety of populations. We will discuss adaptive capacity later in this chapter.

Assessments of Relative Mastery

Researchers have measured relative mastery primarily through quasi-experimental design outcome studies in adult rehabilitation settings. Populations have included individuals post-hip fracture (Buddenberg & Schkade, 1998; Jackson & Schkade, 2001) and cerebrovascular accident (Gibson & Schkade, 1997; Johnson & Schkade, 2001). Of these studies, only two reported using an instrument to standardize intervention. Buddenberg and Schkade (1998) referenced using the Occupational Adaptation Interview Guide designed to help participants determine goals for intervention. Goals identified in the interview led to client-centered occupational therapy interventions to improve relative mastery. Similarly, Stelter and Whisner (2007), reported using the Assessment of Relative Mastery in Occupational Roles (ARMOR), a facility-based assessment to place prisoners in a work program. Although referred to as an assessment of relative mastery, results were not reported because only the instrument's prosocial and antisocial continuum had been subjected to an evaluation of validity. Therefore, to date, no standardized instrument has been used to operationalize interventions in studies designed to improve relative mastery. Instead, researchers' theoretical reasoning has served as the basis of intervention, taking into consideration clients' roles, occupational environments, and personally meaningful goals (Jackson & Schkade, 2001; Johnson, 2006; Johnson & Schkade, 2001).

Results of quantitative studies support improvement in relative mastery of recipients of intervention as measured by a variety of outcome measures. Dependent variables for these studies have included relative mastery (Buddenberg & Schkade, 1998; Gibson & Schkade, 1997; Stelter & Whisner, 2007), functional independence (Buddenberg & Schkade, 1998; Gibson & Schkade, 1997; Jackson & Schkade, 2001; Johannson & Bjorklund, 2005; Johnson & Schkade, 2001), mobility (Johnson & Schkade, 2001), discharge to a least restrictive environment (Buddenberg & Schkade, 1998; Jackson & Schkade, 2001), and length of stay in the facility (Gibson & Schkade, 1997; Jackson & Schkade, 2001). Although improvement in relative mastery has been reported, many tools used in these studies lack standardization and evidence of validity and reliability.

Outcome studies that included descriptive and qualitative methods demonstrated changes in relative mastery for homeless individuals (Johnson, 2006), prisoners (Stelter & Whisner, 2007), and clients post-stroke (Johnson & Schkade, 2001). Descriptive data and example quotes provided support for changes in relative mastery. Johnson and Schkade (2001) reported results of rehabilitation interventions designed to evaluate improvement in mobility and occupational adaptation for three clients post-stroke. Quantitative and qualitative data in this study provided support for improvement in mobility and relative mastery. Increased initiation was demonstrated through clients' participation in activities they have not done for a long time (pp. 102-103). Generalization by these clients post-stroke was evidenced by participants trying activities they had not attempted prior to their participation in the research. One example included a client independently getting out of bed in the middle of the night to check on her husband (p. 103).

Effectiveness, efficiency, and satisfaction to self and others are hallmarks of increased relative mastery (Schkade & Schultz, 2003). Grajo (2017, p. 297) defined the following terms as adapted from Schkade and McClung (2001):

- **Effective participation** in occupations is determined based on how well people achieve the goals of occupational engagement and participation.
- **Efficiency** is people's good use of available resources in the occupational environment (e.g., time, energy, task objects and materials, social supports).
- **Satisfaction** is the extent to which people are content with their occupational performance and the congruence between occupational participation and performance expectations.

Pasek and Schkade (1996) reported that adolescents with limb deficiencies who participated in a 6-day adaptive ski trip demonstrated changes in relative mastery as measured by changes in effectiveness, efficiency, and satisfaction. Improved skill level, increased instructor ratings, and advancement to more difficult slopes are examples of improvement in skiers' effectiveness. Increases in fluid motion and therefore improved performance time were interpreted as increased efficiency because skiers demonstrated new and modified adaptive responses to the challenges of the activity. Increased satisfaction was supported through skier, ski instructor, and observer ratings.

Assessment Tools That Measure Relative Mastery

The Occupational Adaptation Practice Guide (OAPG) was developed to standardize application of the OA model in practice and research (Boone & George-Paschal, 2017). The instrument, previously the Occupational Adaptation Interview Guide (Buddenberg & Schkade, 1998), facilitates occupational therapists to engage clients in the process of identifying occupational challenges and clarifying personal and environmental factors that contribute to and detract from their optimal occupational performance. The instrument also promotes collaboration of the therapist and client in generating relevant goals and specific occupational behaviors to achieve them.

The Relative Mastery Measurement Scale (RMMS; George, Schkade, & Ishee, 2004) is a dichotomous 12-item standardized measure of relative mastery. It was designed to be used by any person, with or without a diagnosis, to evaluate his or her own occupational responses to self-identified challenges. Lu's coefficient of agreement, calculated for five OA experts, was .95 ($P < .05$) supporting the content validity of the measure. Researchers evaluated the RMMS for construct validity using Rasch analysis. Based on pilot data for 142 participants in rehabilitation, a score below five indicated a perception of poor relative mastery. Readers should refer to George et al. (2004) for complete results and a thorough explanation of Rasch analysis. Research is underway that explores the unidimensionality and sensitivity to change for a six-item version of the RMMS. The modified RMMS utilizes a five-point independent scale (-2 to +2). The new measure also provides a mechanism for plotting negative (-2, -1), neutral (0) and positive (+1, +2) relative mastery ratings on an x-y axis. The OAPG is also being used in research to standardize application of the OA theory.

The Family Looking Into Family Experiences (L.I.F.E) is an occupation-based assessment for use with families who have a child diagnosed with autism spectrum disorder (Honaker, Rosello, & Candler, 2012). Based on the OA model, the instrument facilitates a collaborative dialogue between the therapist and a family member to "identify, evaluate, and measure perceived success in unique and relevant family occupations" (p. 618).

The instrument includes time diaries, inquiries about routines and rituals, and the family member's rating of their perceived relative mastery for five family-selected occupations (effectiveness, efficiency, and satisfaction). A study of test-retest reliability of the Family L.I.F.E. was implemented with a sample of 13 families (Honaker et al., 2012). Nonparametric results with 1 week between administrations revealed strong positive relationships for effectiveness and satisfaction questions and moderate positive relationships for efficiency questions.

OCCUPATIONAL IDENTITY AND OCCUPATIONAL COMPETENCE AS AN INDICATOR OF OCCUPATIONAL ADAPTATION

The Model of Human Occupation (MOHO) defines occupational adaptation as a mechanism of "constructing a positive occupational identity and achieving occupational competence over time in the context of one's environment" (Kielhofner, 2008, p. 107). Occupational adaptation is critical in allowing the person to gather a sense of who he or she is as an occupational being (occupational identity) and identify the extent to which he or she has a sustained pattern of occupational performance and participation (occupational competence) (Clifford-O'Brien, 2017). For a more detailed focus on occupational adaptation as defined within the MOHO, refer to Chapter 6 of this text.

Numerous researchers have qualitatively explored occupational adaptation with thematic results focused on the adaptation of the person, modification of occupations, and occupational identity relative to a personal choice or disability. A variety of populations living with the effects of an injury or illness have been studied, including individuals who have sustained a traumatic brain injury (Hoogerdijk, Runge, & Haugboelle, 2011; Klinger, 2005; Parsons & Stanley, 2008; Soeker, 2011), multiple sclerosis (MS; Cahill, Connolly, & Stapleton, 2010; Lexell, Iwarsson, & Lund, 2011), trauma recovery (Precin, 2011), long-term illness (Johansson & Isaksson, 2011), and heart failure (Norberg, Boman, Löfgren, & Brännström, 2014). Research has also been conducted for participants who have engaged in the occupation of smoking cessation (Luck & Beagan, 2015), persons who experienced religious or spiritual conflict due to their identification as lesbian, gay, bisexual, transgender, or queer (LGBTQ; Beagan & Hattie, 2015), and college students in Jordan who experienced conflicts between their values and cultural expectations (Yazdani, 2011). Thematic results of these studies have demonstrated the complexity of participants' engagement in challenging occupations, occupational identity, and occupational adaptation. The same process of adaptation appears evident across studies, without regard to whether participants were experiencing a physical disability, volitionally attempting to stop smoking, or experiencing a conflict of identity. First, challenges to one's occupational performance creates an occupational disruption leading to difficulty in maintaining or developing a new positive occupational identity. Second, participants attempt to successfully perform relevant occupations leading to either reinforcement of or a change in their identity, modification of aspects of the activity, or creation of new patterns of occupational performance. Third, occupational identity and occupational adaptation either improved or the transition resulted in an awareness of losses, or some of both.

Acknowledging the complexity of the occupational adaptation process, Luck and Beagan (2015) and Nayar and Stanley (2015) suggested there is a need for further investigation into the interaction between occupational identity and occupational adaptation. Differences of opinion exist in the literature related to which comes first: changes in occupational identity or occupational adaptation. Klinger (2005) stated that changes in occupational identity preceded successful adaptation in occupation. In contrast, Soeker (2011), Hoogerdijk et al. (2011), and Parsons and Stanley (2008), who also conducted research with individuals post-brain injury, asserted that it was the struggle of engaging in routine occupations that ultimately facilitated occupational adaptation that led to participants' new identities. Luck and Beagan (2015) discovered that adopting the identity of nonsmoker helped a sample of adults achieve their voluntary transition from smoker to nonsmoker. Competency and ultimately their changed identity was attributed, in part, to their repeated attempts to stop smoking. The authors discussed the complex interaction that existed between occupational identity and occupational adaptation for these participants. Luck and Beagan (2015) also suggested that there is a need to learn more about possible differences in the occupational adaptation process when transitions are voluntary versus those that are nonvoluntary.

Lexell et al. (2011) highlighted the importance of knowing a consumer's stage in the adaptation process for client-centered practice. They emphasized that occupational therapy interventions must be consistent with the consumer's own occupational identity. Without this knowledge, they asserted that an occupational therapist may invalidly focus therapy on modifying activities when the client is still attempting to "preserve his/her previous capable self" and is not ready to "adapt occupations to live with a changed sense of self" (p. 132). Being sensitive to the client's stage in the adaptation process allows him or her to remain the expert in his or her readiness for adaptation. Norberg et al. (2014) reported that when the time was right, research participants with congestive heart failure redefined their life with consideration to their new limitations and adjusted their occupations accordingly. The ability to adapt is often complicated by the lack of available physical, social, and cultural support from the environment.

Assessment Tools That Measure Occupational Identity and Occupational Competence

The majority of research related to occupational identity and occupational competency have employed qualitative methodologies to generate knowledge. However, Cahill et al. (2010) incorporated four standardized semi-structured interviews based on MOHO as part of their inquiry into the impact of the diagnosis of MS on participants as occupational beings. The assessments included the Occupational Performance History Interview II (OPHI II; Kielhofner et al., 2004), the Modified Interest Checklist (Kielhofner & Neville, 1983), the Role Checklist (Oakley, Kielhofner, & Barris, 1985) and the Occupational Questionnaire (Smith, Kielhofner, & Watts, 1986). Descriptive results were used by the researchers to discover patterns in participants' past, present, and future occupations; patterns of engagement; and occupational identity and occupational competence.

Another instrument based on the MOHO and designed as a measure of occupational adaptation is the Occupational Case Analysis Interview and Rating Scale (OCAIRS; Forsyth et al., 2005; Lai, Haglund, & Kielhofner, 1999). The instrument is a 14-item measure rated on a five-point Likert scale by therapists after a semi-structured interview. For a list of other MOHO-based measures related to occupational competence and identity, refer to Chapter 6.

ADAPTIVE CAPACITY AS AN INDICATOR OF OCCUPATIONAL ADAPTATION

Adaptive capacity can be understood using the analogy of "tools in a toolbox" (Grajo, 2017). Adaptive capacity is the person's ability to assess his or her perception for the need to change, modify, or refine a variety of responses to occupational challenges in the environment (Schkade & Schultz, 2003). In Grajo's reconceptualization of Schkade and Schultz's OA model (2017), he offered some questions to qualitatively assess a person's adaptive capacity (p. 297):

- How do you typically respond when faced with such an occupational challenge?
- Do these responses help you overcome the challenge?
- When you find that your usual ways of responding to a challenge do not work, what do you do? What other strategies or responses do you use?
- What responses and strategies do you use that you think are helpful and not helpful when faced with such occupational challenges?
- Do you think you have a good variety of responses and strategies you use when overcoming challenges?

From a neuroscience perspective, adaptive capacity is comparable with adaptive plasticity, described as an "innate ability of the central nervous system to adapt or modify behavioral responses after exposure to a challenge to the system" (Kovic & Schultz-Krohn, 2013, p. 457). Challenges can result from stimuli internal and external to the person. For a more detailed discussion on neural mechanisms supporting occupational adaptation, refer to Chapters 3 and 4. According to Schultz (2014), impairment in adaptive capacity can be experienced as a result of stressful life transitions, including physical disabilities or emotional difficulties.

Numerous researchers have descriptively and qualitatively explored the impact of a variety of transitional impairments. Meta-ethnographic synthesis studies have explored the adaptive capacity of parents of pre-term infants (Gibbs, Boshoff, & Stanley, 2015), individuals who have sustained a stroke (Williams & Murray, 2013a), and those coping after experiencing a hand injury (Bates & Mason, 2014). Outcomes research aimed at evaluating the impact of intervention approaches on adaptive capacity have been conducted by Johansson and Bjorklund (2016) and Whisner, Stelter, and Schultz (2014). Johansson and Bjorklund (2016) evaluated the impact of intervention on older persons' health, well-being, and occupational adaptation. Whisner et al. (2014) evaluated the impact of a change in the environment on participants' rates of engagement in mental health group therapy sessions.

The key factor in facilitating the adaptive capacity of consumers of occupational therapy is the person and environment transaction (Lee et al., 2006; Schultz, 2009; Spencer, Davidson, & White, 1996). Within this transaction, the doing of the person is perceived as essential to his or her adaptation (Schkade & Schultz, 1992). The client's choice of meaningful occupation is also reported to be essential to eliciting the process of adaptation (Grajo, 2017; Schultz, 2014).

Adaptation has been described as individual and situated (Hoogerdijk et al., 2011) and the struggle that occurs during the pursuit of improvement in occupational functioning results from the combination of the person's desires and the demands of the environment (Krusen, 2015; Lee et al., 2006; Schkade & Schultz, 1992; Schultz, 2009). For more about the situated and transactional perspective on occupational adaptation, refer to Chapter 10 of this text. Familiar environments and social supports have been cited as having a positive influence on adaptation (Parsons & Stanley, 2008). Specifically, a sense of belonging and social roles have been associated with adaptation (Gibbs et al., 2015; Johansson & Bjorklund, 2016). The learning that occurs as a result of the interaction between person and environment often contributes to reinforcement of the adaptive process (Luck & Beagan, 2015; Schultz, 2009; Schultz & Schkade, 1992).

Conversely, the inability to participate in occupations may limit adaptive capacity and place individuals at risk for dysadaptation (Beagan & Hattie, 2015; Firefirey & Hess-April, 2014; Krusen, 2015; McDougall, Buchanan, & Peterson, 2014; Peterson et al., 1999; Rudman, Huot, Klinger, Leipert, & Spafford, 2010; Yazdani, 2011). Challenges to adaptive capacity have been described for populations who have made volitional choices to participate in occupations such as smoking cessation (Luck & Beagan, 2015), those who incurred an injury or illness (Firefirey & Hess-April, 2014; Rudman et al., 2010), individuals who experienced an inconsistency between their values and those of their environment (Beagan & Hattie, 2015; Yazdani, 2011), older persons who struggle with a fear of falling (Peterson et al., 1999), primary caregivers for others (McDougall et al., 2014), and occupational therapy fieldwork students (Krusen, 2015).

Emotions that have been used to explain participants' perceived need or demand for adaptation include shock (Williams & Murray, 2013b), helplessness (Ammann, Satink, & Andresen, 2012), restricted engagement (McDougall et al., 2014), increased sense of risk (Rudman et al., 2010), loss of self (Johansson & Isaksson, 2011; Soeker, 2011), necessary struggle (Hoogerdijk et al., 2011), panic (Pepin & Deutscher, 2011), conflict (Beagan & Hattie, 2015; Yazdani, 2011), feeling invisible (Pepin & Deutscher, 2011), disruption (Gibbs et al., 2015; Rosenfield, 1989), and difficulty navigating the environment (Williams & Murray, 2013a, 2013b). Consistent with the notion of activation, as described in the OA model (Schultz, 2014), these emotional reactions required participants to draw upon their adaptive capacity.

From an awareness of failure or risk, individuals are often afforded opportunities to make conscious choices to overcome their personal challenges (Krusen, 2015; Nayar & Stanley, 2015), learn (Luck & Beagan, 2015), grow and engage in meaningful occupations (Hoogerdijk et al., 2011; Johansson & Bjorklund, 2016; Precin, 2011; Soeker, 2011), explore new opportunities (Precin, 2011), establish routines (Nayar & Stanley,

2015), maintain and reclaim roles (Gibbs et al., 2015), engage in new roles (Pepin & Deutscher, 2011), increase cognitive planning (Williams & Murray, 2013b); strive for independence (Rudman et al., 2010), limit environments that place them at risk (Rudman et al., 2010), engage in familiar environments (Hoogerdijk et al., 2011), and resume activities with modification (Ammann et al., 2012; Bates & Mason, 2014; Norberg et al., 2014; Williams & Murray, 2013a).

Participant groups shared that they have learned to modify or change interests (Cahill et al., 2010; Nayar & Stanley, 2015; Williams & Murray, 2013a), modify their time and tempo (Johansson & Isaksson, 2011), live a changed family life (Lexell et al., 2011), and do activities together with others (Bates & Mason, 2014; Lee et al., 2006). Descriptions of the adaptation process have often included one or more of the following strategies: modifying occupations, accepting help, avoiding occupations (Ammann et al., 2012; Bates & Mason, 2014; Luck & Beagan, 2015; Williams & Murray, 2013b), and adapting the environment (Norberg et al., 2014).

Researchers have suggested that occupational therapists, to facilitate an increase in clients' adaptive capacities, should prepare individuals for future transitions (Hersch et al., 2012; Pepin & Deutscher, 2011); consider the significant role of valued occupations in adaptation (Bates & Mason, 2014; Firefirey & Hess-April, 2014; Johansson & Bjorklund, 2016; Lexell et al., 2011); provide environments that create social support for participation in roles (Johansson & Bjorklund, 2016; Whisner et al., 2014); use humor, human touch, and expression of anger and promote positive self-talk and hope (Williams & Murray, 2013b); consider the adaptation phase of the person (Lexell et al., 2011); and incorporate conscious choice on the part of the client (Nayar & Stanley, 2015). They have also suggested that occupational therapists should utilize a more process-oriented approach than one that is performance-driven (Hoogerdijk et al., 2011).

ADVANCING THE KNOWLEDGE ON OCCUPATIONAL ADAPTATION

Results of quantitative, qualitative, and mixed-methods research have meaningfully contributed to our profession's comprehensive understanding of the construct of occupational adaptation as a measure of occupational participation. The authors propose that future research efforts increase in quantitative and mixed methods to provide an evaluation of the efficacy of theory-based approaches aimed to improve occupational adaptation. Researchers are encouraged to use valid and reliable measures to scientifically evaluate outcomes of intervention approaches that aim to improve occupational adaptation. The development of instruments guided by occupation-based models with a clear articulation of the construct of occupational adaptation and tested for psychometric properties is also essential.

This chapter has presented an overview of how the construct of occupational adaptation has been assessed in the occupational therapy literature. Although references have been made in this chapter to theories and research traditions, this synthesized review of the occupational therapy literature transcends theoretical orientation and research methodologies. Whether the focus of the research is on relative mastery, occupational identity and occupational competence, or adaptive capacity, the ultimate goal is the achievement of occupational adaptation. A common theme of the studies reviewed was that choosing and engaging in meaningful occupations facilitates occupational adaptation while barriers and limitations to participation inhibit or restrict adaptation. This appears to be the case whether individuals volitionally chose a transition or had a challenge thrust upon them by an injury or illness, or whether it resulted from their interaction with their physical, social, or cultural environment. The actual act of "doing" was consistently associated with improved occupational adaptation, as evidenced by increased relative mastery, initiation, and generalization; occupational identity and occupational competence; adaptive capacity; and adaptive responses and strategies. Future research should evaluate the efficacy of theory-based protocols aimed at increasing occupational adaptation, investigate the complexities of the relationship between the various indicators of occupational adaptation, and compare outcomes of the timing and intensity of interventions for various populations.

SUMMARY AND IMPLICATIONS

- Occupational adaptation can be defined as an outcome of occupational participation.
- The construct of occupational adaptation can be measured through quantitative and qualitative methods.
- Impacts on relative mastery, occupational identity and competence, and adaptive capacity are some ways of describing the impact of occupational therapy intervention on the occupational adaptation process of clients or the impact of OA-guided intervention.
- There are published tools that can be used to measure occupational adaptation. Researchers are encouraged to develop more tools guided by occupational adaptation principles and determine the psychometric properties of these tools.

REFERENCES

Ammann, B., Satink, T., & Andresen, M. (2012) Experiencing occupations with chronic hand disabilities: Narratives of hand-injured adults. *Hand Therapy, 17*(4), 87-94.

Asher, I. E. (2014). *Asher's occupational therapy assessment tools: An annotated index* (4th ed.). Bethesda, MD: AOTA.

Bates, E., & Mason, R. (2014). Coping strategies used by people with a major hand injury: A review of the literature. *British Journal of Occupational Therapy, 77*(6), 289-295.

Beagan, B. L., & Hattie, B. (2015). LGBTQ experiences with religion and spirituality: Occupational transition and adaptation. *Journal of Occupational Science, 22*(4), 459-476. doi:10.1080/14427591.2014.9 53670

Boone, A., & George-Paschal, L. (2017) Feasibility testing of the Occupational Adaptation Practice Guide. *British Journal of Occupational Therapy, 80*(6), 368-374.

Buddenberg, L. A., & Schkade, J. K. (1998). Special feature: A comparison of occupational therapy intervention approaches for older patients after hip fracture. *Topics in Geriatric Rehabilitation, 13*(4), 52-68.

Cahill, M., Connolly, D., & Stapleton, T. (2010). Exploring occupational adaptation through the lives of women with multiple sclerosis. *British Journal of Occupational Therapy, 73*(3), 106-115.

Clifford-O'Brien, J. (2017). Model of human occupation. In J. Hinojosa, P. Kramer, & C. Royeen (Eds.), *Perspectives on human occupation: Theories underlying practice* (2nd ed., pp. 93-136). Philadelphia, PA: F.A. Davis.

Doucet, B. M., & Gutman, S. A. (2013). Quantifying function: The rest of the measurement story. *American Journal of Occupational Therapy, 67*, 7-9.

Firefirey, N., & Hess-April, L. (2014). A study to explore occupational adaptation of adults with MDR-TB who undergo long-term hospitalization. *South African Journal of Occupational Therapy, 44*(3), 18-23.

Forsyth, K., Deshpande, S., Kielhofner, G., Hendriksson, C., Haglund, L., Olson, L., … Kulkarni, S. (2005). Occupational Circumstances Assessment Interview Rating Scale (OCAIRS), Version 4. In I. E. Asher (Ed.), *Asher's occupational therapy assessment tools: An annotated index* (pp. 47-48).

George, L. A., Schkade, J. K., & Ishee, J. H. (2004). Content validity of the Relative Mastery Measurement Scale: A measure of occupational adaptation. *OTJR: Occupation, Participation and Health, 24*(3), 92-102.

Gibbs, D., Boshoff, K., & Stanley, M. (2015). Becoming the parent of a preterm infant: A meta-ethnographic synthesis. *British Journal of Occupational Therapy, 78*(8), 475-487.

Gibson, J. W., & Schkade, J. K. (1997). Occupational adaptation intervention with patients with cerebrovascular accident: A clinical study. *American Journal of Occupational Therapy, 51*(7), 523-529.

Grajo, L. (2017). Occupational adaptation. In J. Hinojosa, P. Kramer, & C. Royeen (Eds.), *Perspectives on human occupation: Theories underlying practice* (2nd ed., pp. 287-311). Philadelphia, PA: F.A. Davis.

Hersch, G., Hutchinson, S., Davidson, H., Wilson, C., Maharaj, T., & Watson, K. B. (2012). Effect of an occupation-based cultural heritage intervention in long-term geriatric care: A two-group control study. *American Journal of Occupational Therapy, 66*(2), 224-232.

Honaker, D., Rosello, S., & Candler, C. (2012). Test-retest reliability of Family L.I.F.E. (looking into family experiences): An occupation-based assessment. *American Journal of Occupational Therapy, 66*(5), 617-620.

Hoogerdijk, B., Runge, U., & Haugboelle, J. (2011). The adaptation process after traumatic brain injury: An individual and ongoing occupational struggle to gain a new identity. *Scandinavian Journal of Occupational Therapy, 18*, 122-132.

Jackson, J. P., & Schkade, J. K. (2001). Occupational adaptation model versus biomechanical-rehabilitation model in the treatment of patients with hip fractures. *American Journal of Occupational Therapy, 55*(5), 531-537.

Johansson, A., & Bjorklund, A. (2005). Occupational adaptation or well-tried, professional experience in rehabilitation of the disabled elderly at home. *Activities, Adaptations & Aging, 30*, 1-21.

Johansson, A., & Bjorklund, A. (2016). The impact of occupational therapy and lifestyle interventions on older persons' health, well-being, and occupational adaptation. *Scandinavian Journal of Occupational Therapy, 23*(3), 207-219.

Johansson, C., & Isaksson, G. (2011). Experiences of participation in occupations of women on long-term sick leave. *Scandinavian Journal of Occupational Therapy, 18*(4), 294-301. doi:10.3109/11038128.2010.521950

Johnson, J. A. (2006). Describing the phenomenon of homelessness through the theory of occupational adaptation. *Occupational Therapy in Health Care, 20*, 63-80. doi:10.1080/J003v20n03_05

Johnson, J. A., & Schkade, J. K. (2001). Effects of an occupation-based intervention on mobility problems following a cerebral vascular accident. *Journal of Applied Gerontology, 20*(1), 91-110.

Kielhofner, G. (2008). *Model of human occupation: Theory and application* (4th ed.). Philadelphia, PA: Lippincott Williams & Wilkins.

Kielhofner, G., Mallinson, T., Crawford, C., Nowak, M., Rigby, M., Henry, A., & Walens, D. (2004). *Occupational Performance History Interview–II (OPHI-II), Version 2.* Chicago, IL: Model of Human Occupation Clearing House, Department of Occupational Therapy, College of Applied Sciences, University of Illinois.

Kielhofner, G., & Neville, A. (1983). *The Modified Interest Checklist.* Unpublished manuscript, University of Illinois at Chicago, Chicago, IL.

Klinger, L. (2005). Occupational adaptation: Perspectives of people with traumatic brain injury. *Journal of Occupational Science 1*, 9-16. doi:10.1080/14427591.2005.9686543

Kovic, M., & Schultz-Krohn, W. (2013). *Performance skills: Definitions and evaluation in the context of the Occupational Therapy Framework.* St. Louis, MO: Elsevier.

Krusen, N. E. (2015). Student voices of adaptation following fieldwork failure. *International Journal of Practice-Based Learning in Health and Social Care, 3*(1), 16-29.

Lai, J. S., Haglund, L., & Kielhofner, G. (1999). Occupational case analysis interview and rating scale: An examination of construct validity. *Scandinavian Journal of Caring Science, 13,* 267-273.

Lee, M., Madden, V., Mason, K., Rice, S., Wyburd, J., & Hobson, S. (2006). Occupational engagement and adaptation in adults with dementia: A preliminary investigation. *Physical and Occupational Therapy and Geriatrics, 25*(1), 63-81.

Lexell, E. M., Iwarsson, S., & Lund, M. L. (2011). Occupational adaptation in people with multiple sclerosis. *OTJR: Occupation, Participation and Health, 31*(3), 127-134.

Luck, K., & Beagan, B. (2015). Occupational transition of smoking cessation in women: "You're restructuring your whole life." *Journal of Occupational Science, 22*(2), 183-196. doi:10.1080/14427591.2014 .887418

McDougall, C., Buchanan, A., & Peterson, S. (2014). Understanding primary carers' occupational adaptation and engagement. *Australian Journal of Occupational Therapy, 61,* 83-91.

Nayar, S., & Stanley, M. (2015). Occupational adaptation as a social process in everyday life. *Journal of Occupational Science, 22*(1), 26-38.

Norberg, E. B., Boman, K., Löfgren, B., & Brännström, M. (2014). Occupational performance and strategies for managing daily life among the elderly with heart failure. *Scandinavian Journal of Occupational Therapy, 21*(5), 392-399. doi:10.3109/11038128.2014.911955

Oakley, F., Kielhofner, G., & Barris, R. (1985). An occupational therapy approach to assessing psychiatric patients' adaptive functioning. *American Journal of Occupational Therapy, 39,* 147-154.

Parsons, L., & Stanley, M. (2008). The lived experience of occupational adaptation following acquired brain injury for people living in the rural area. *Australian Occupational Therapy Journal, 55,* 231-328.

Pasek, P. B., & Schkade, J. K. (1996). Effects of a skiing experience on adolescents with limb deficiencies: An occupational adaptation perspective. *American Journal of Occupational Therapy, 50*(1), 24-31.

Pepin, G., & Deutscher, B. (2011). The lived experience of Australian retirees: 'I'm retired, what do I do now?' *British Journal of Occupational Therapy, 74*(9), 419-426.

Peterson, E., Howland, J., Kielhofner, G., Lachman, M. E., Assmann, S., Cote, J., & Jett, A. (1999). Falls self-efficacy and occupational adaptation among elders. *Physical & Occupational Therapy in Geriatrics, 16*(1-2), 1-16. doi:10.1080/J148v16n01_01

Precin, P. (2011). Occupation as therapy for trauma recovery: A case study. *Work, 38*(1), 78-81. doi:10.3233/ WOR-2011-1106

Rosenfield, M. S. (1989). Occupational disruption and adaptation: A study of house fire victims. *American Journal of Occupational Therapy, 43*(2), 89-96.

Rudman, D. L., Huot, S., Klinger, L., Leipert, B. D., & Spafford, M. M. (2010). Struggling to maintain occupation while dealing with risk: The experiences of older adults with low vision. *OTJR: Occupation, Participation and Health, 30*(2), 87-96.

Schkade, J., & McClung, M. (2001). *Occupational adaptation in practice: Concepts and cases.* Thorofare, NJ: SLACK Incorporated.

Schkade, J. K., & Schultz, S. (1992). Occupational Adaptation: Toward a holistic approach for contemporary practice. Part I. *American Journal of Occupational Therapy, 46*(9), 829-837.

Schkade, J. K., & Schultz, S. (2003). Occupational adaptation. In P. Kramer, J. Hinojosa, & C. B. Royeen (Eds.), *Perspectives in human occupation: Participation in life* (pp. 181-221). Baltimore, MD: Lippincott Williams & Wilkins.

Schultz, S. (2009). Theory of occupational adaptation. In E. B. Crepeau, E. S. Cohn, & B. A. Boyt Schell (Eds.), *Williard and Spackman's occupational therapy* (11th ed.). Philadelphia, PA: Lippincott Williams & Wilkins.

Schultz, S. (2014). Theory of occupational adaptation. In B. A. Boyt Schell, G. Gillen, M.E. Scaffa, & E. S. Cohn (Eds.), *Williard and Spackman's occupational therapy* (12th ed.). Philadelphia, PA: Lippincott Williams & Wilkins.

Schultz, S., & Schkade, J. K. (1992). Occupational adaptation: Toward a holistic approach for contemporary practice, part 2. *American Journal of Occupational Therapy, 46*(10), 917-925. doi:10.5014/ajot.46.10.917

Smith, N., Kielhofner, G., & Watts, J. (1986). The relationship between volition, activity pattern and life satisfaction in the elderly. *American Journal of Occupational Therapy, 40,* 278-283.

Soeker, M. S. (2011). Occupational adaptation: A return to work perspective of persons with mild to moderate brain injury in South Africa. *Journal of Occupational Science, 18*(1), 81-91.

Spencer, J. C., Davidson, H. A., & White, V. K. (1996). Continuity and change: Past experience as adaptive repertoire in occupational adaptation. *American Journal of Occupational Therapy, 50*(7), 526-534.

Stelter, L., & Whisner, S. M. (2007). Building responsibility for self through meaningful roles. *Occupational Therapy in Mental Health, 23*(1), 69-84. doi:10.1300/J004v23n01_05

Whisner, S. M., Stelter, L. D., & Schultz, S. (2014). Influence of three interventions on group participation in an acute psychiatric facility. *Occupational Therapy in Mental Health, 30*, 26-42. doi:10.1080/0164 212X.2014.878527

Williams, S., & Murray, C. (2013a). The experience of engaging in occupation following stroke: A qualitative meta-synthesis. *British Journal of Occupational Therapy, 76*(8), 370-378.

Williams, S., & Murray, C. (2013b). Lived experiences of older adults' occupational adaptation following stroke. *Australian Occupational Therapy Journal, 60*, 39-47.

Yazdani, F. (2011). How students with low level subjective wellbeing perceive the impact of the environment on occupational behavior. *International Journal of Therapy and Rehabilitation, 18*(8), 462-470.

Section II

NEUROSCIENCE PERSPECTIVES ON OCCUPATIONAL ADAPTATION

Angela K. Boisselle, PhD, OTR, ATP and Lenin C. Grajo, PhD, EdM, OTR/L

OVERVIEW

In Section II, we explore the underlying neurological, cognitive, and behavioral influences of adaptation. Chapter 3 provides a synthesis of neuroscience and movement science literature as a basis to developmental, synaptic, and functional neuroplasticity that influence typical human adaptation. Studies from pediatric and adult populations in rehabilitation medicine and neuroscience provide potential supporting evidence for the core definition of occupational adaptation. The chapter provides examples of evidence-based practice from adult and pediatric research that demonstrate recovery of function following an injury as evidenced by changes in the brain, transaction with the environment, and engagement in occupation.

Chapter 4 presents a synthesis of literature from behavioral and cognitive neuroscience based on the foundational aspects of neuroscience presented in Chapter 3. Specifically, we examine complex neurobiological aspects of the brain that influence the internal processes of motivation, intentional and goal-directed behaviors, and resilience. Examples of clinical evidence are presented related to occupational adaptation in a variety of pediatric and adult issues such as substance abuse, trauma, developmental disorders, adverse life events, and post-traumatic stress disorders. The chapter explores the possibility that the use of the cognitive and behavioral internal processes promote participation in functional tasks and occupations and is ultimately necessary to support health, wellness, and adaptation.

Both chapters offer a case story that exemplify the value of understanding underlying neurological processes in the recovery and process of occupational adaptation.

3

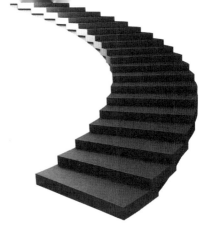

Neural Basis of Adaptation
Neuroplasticity and Movement Sciences

Dawn M. Nilsen, EdD, OTR/L, FAOTA and
Angela K. Boisselle, PhD, OTR, ATP

OVERVIEW The connection between neuroscience and the construct of occupational adaptation has not been extensively studied. This is evident in literature presented in Chapters 1 and 2. The authors' intent for this chapter is to challenge the reader to frame occupational adaptation as a process that occurs at the neurocellular level.

Neurological adaptation is a complex and dynamic process, commonly referred to as *neuroplasticity*. During human development, synaptic connectivity begins, and this connectivity is modified throughout the course of life as a consequence of the interplay between genetic factors and the child's transaction with the environment. This adaptability of the nervous system continues throughout the life span and involves changes ranging from modifications in synaptic efficacy to lasting structural and functional changes reflected in the numbers and types of connections among neurons within brain regions and between brain regions. These neuronal changes serve as the basis of occupational adaptation, underlying motor learning, memory, and the recovery of function after neurologic injury.

Grajo LC, Boisselle AK, eds.
Adaptation Through Occupation:
Multidimensional Perspectives (pp 35-57).
© 2019 SLACK Incorporated.

CHAPTER OBJECTIVES By the end of this chapter, the reader will be able to:
- Describe the structures and function of neurons and neuronal communication significant for neuroplasticity.
- Define neuroplasticity and differentiate the types that occur as a result of development, experience, injury or disease in typical development, and a disease process.
- Synthesize research that provides evidence of the likely neural mechanisms associated with occupational adaptation.
- Describe pediatric and adult client population research, which illustrates the neuroplastic mechanisms that are influenced by engagement in occupation and promote recovery of function.

QUESTIONS FOR DISCUSSION AND REFLECTION As the reader explores this chapter, let the following questions guide discussion and reflection:
- How will knowledge of neural structures aid me in understanding the process of adaptation in my clients as a result of disability, illness, or disruption of typical human development?
- How can I articulate and apply the process of adaptation using knowledge on neuroplasticity?

INTRODUCTION

Occupational adaptation is a transactional process that occurs when an individual is faced with diversity or change and they attempt to produce a response that results in mastery over that challenge (Grajo, 2017). This internal process will result in structural and functional changes in the brain, known as *neuroplasticity*. The brain physically changes in response to development, experience, and/or damage or dysfunction. Neuroplasticity can be described at various levels within the nervous system and occurs, with varying capacity, throughout the life span. For the purposes of this chapter, we will examine neuroplasticity in terms of adaptation and how participation in occupation influences changes in the brain. To begin, a brief overview of neurons, synaptic transmission, and the basics of neuronal communication illustrating the differences between neuronal circuits that underlie simple forms of adaptation versus more complex forms of adaptation will set the foundation for this chapter and Chapter 4. This will be followed by a synthesis of neuroscience and motor learning literature depicting the neural mechanisms that underlie the normative process of occupational adaptation. Finally, the chapter will highlight research conducted with pediatric and adult client populations that illustrate neuroplastic mechanisms that underlie recovery of function after injury or disease that result from engagement in occupation.

NEURONS AND NEURONAL COMMUNICATION

The neuron is the structural and functional unit of the nervous system. Neurons detect changes in the environment, integrate and communicate this information to other

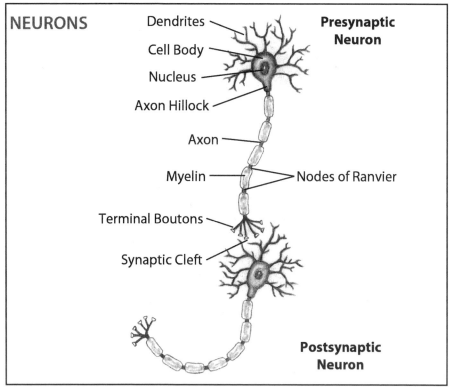

NEURONS

Dendrites

Cell Body

Nucleus

Axon Hillock

Axon

Myelin — Nodes of Ranvier

Terminal Boutons

Synaptic Cleft

Presynaptic Neuron

Postsynaptic Neuron

Figure 3-1. The neuron. (Reprinted with permission from Gutman, S. [2017]. *Quick reference neuroscience for rehabilitation professionals: The essential neurologic principles underlying rehabilitation practice* [3rd ed.]. Thorofare, NJ: SLACK Incorporated.)

neurons, and control the bodily responses that allow us to interact with our environment in effective and efficient ways. Therefore, any type of behavioral response, whether simple or complex, involves information transfer between neurons, also known as *neuronal communication*. Neurons communicate by converting electrical signals into chemical signals, which are then converted back to electrical signals. These signals can be excitatory or inhibitory, creating complex patterns of activity in neuronal circuits or networks that are at the heart of occupational adaptation. Although it is not the purpose of this chapter to provide a full account of the structure and function of neurons or neuronal communication, brief overviews of the important features of a typical neuron, synaptic transmission, and communication in neuronal circuits are provided for context.

Structure of a Typical Neuron

A typical neuron consists of a soma (cell body), dendrites, and an axon, and the inside of the neuron is separated from its outside cellular environment by a membrane called the *neuronal membrane* (Figure 3-1). Each feature of the neuron plays a unique role in its ability to serve as the communicator of the nervous system. The soma contains the organelles of the cell and is where gene expression, gene transcription, and protein synthesis occurs. The axons are considered the sending end of the neuron. The axon and its branches allow for the transmission of information, in the form of an electrical signal, over long distances throughout multiple parts of the nervous system. Each axon ends at what is known as the axon terminal, which contains synaptic vesicles that contain neurotransmitters. *Neurotransmitters* are the chemical signals that the brain uses to transmit information.

The site where an axon terminal comes in contact with another neuron is called the *synapse*. Many synapses occur at the point of contact between an axon terminal of one neuron and the dendrites of another neuron. Thus, dendrites are considered the receiving end of the neuron. Neurons have various numbers of dendritic branches, which are often covered with structures called *dendritic spines*. The *neuronal membrane* surrounds the dendrites, and dendritic spines contain multiple receptor proteins that serve as the binding sites for neurotransmitters. The neuronal membrane holds an electrical potential at rest, and it is changes in this potential that cause electrical current flow in neurons.

Overview of Synaptic Transmission

The synapse is the location where information is transferred from one neuron to another, and this transfer of information is known as *synaptic transmission*. Synaptic transmission can be excitatory or inhibitory. The synapse consists of a presynaptic side and a postsynaptic side. The presynaptic side is formed by the axon terminal of the sending (i.e., presynaptic) neuron, and the postsynaptic side is usually formed by the dendrite or soma of the receiving (i.e., postsynaptic) neuron. The space between the presynaptic and postsynaptic neuron is called the *synaptic cleft*. Neurotransmitters released in response to an electrical impulse from the presynaptic neuron traverse the cleft and bind receptors embedded on the surface of the membrane of the postsynaptic neuron. The binding of a neurotransmitter to its receptor causes a change in the neuronal membrane potential; consequently, the chemical signal is converted back into an electrical signal, and information transmission continues, allowing neurons to communicate with each other.

Overview of Neuronal Circuits

The description of synaptic transmission illustrates how one presynaptic neuron communicates with one postsynaptic neuron; however, neurons communicate with each other in circuits that vary in complexity. For example, some circuits form functional links between the brain and spinal cord that modulate reflexive responses to sensory stimuli, whereas other circuits form functional links within and between brain regions, forming complex neuronal networks that work together to mediate higher-level functions such as motor planning, motor learning, and memory formation.

To illustrate the concept of communication in neuronal circuits, let us consider the adaptive behavioral response of pulling one's hand away from a hot stove during a cooking activity. When we touch something hot, sensory neurons in our skin perceive the noxious thermal information. In turn, they excite motor neurons, which activate the muscles that allow us to withdraw our hand from the hot surface. This sensory information is also conveyed to the somatosensory cortex, allowing us to localize the painful stimulus. This is an example of a simple circuit in which excitation in the upstream neuron (sensory neuron) is fed forward through the neuronal chain in a way that propagates excitation in the downstream neurons (i.e., flexor motor neurons and somatosensory neurons). Conversely, a circuit that feeds forward inhibition results in the shutting down or limiting of excitation in the downstream neurons. For example, in order for a smooth flexor withdrawal response to take place in the previous example, antagonist muscles in the upper limb must decrease their activity. Feed-forward inhibition in a circuit will allow this to happen (Byrne, n.d.).

Furthermore, a single neuron can receive input from thousands of presynaptic neurons and that neuron can in turn communicate with thousands of postsynaptic neurons. This is known as convergence and divergence, respectively. *Convergence* allows a neuron to receive multiple inputs from many other neurons in a network and *divergence* allows one neuron to communicate with multiple neurons in a network (Byrne, n.d.). The processes of convergence and divergence allows for complex integration and transfer of information between many sources. In our example, it is likely that touching the hot stove stimulated multiple sensory neurons. Likewise, in order to produce a smooth flexor withdrawal of the hand, multiple motor neurons would need to be activated, whereas antagonist muscle groups would need to be relaxed. Thus, at the neural level, convergence and divergence lead to activation of feed-forward excitation and feed-forward inhibition circuits that mediate the adaptive behavioral response of pulling one's hand away from a hot stove. Of course, this example depicts a very simple adaptive behavior. More complex behavioral adaptations (e.g., performing our morning self-care routine, driving, or playing the piano) will involve simultaneous activation of distinct modular neural networks located in various regions of the brain (e.g., sensorimotor cortices, auditory cortices, and visual cortices). It is the cooperative activation of these functional modules that allow us to engage successfully within our environment and adapt to occupational challenges (Grafman, 2000).

NEUROPLASTICITY AND THE INTERNAL PROCESS OF OCCUPATIONAL ADAPTATION

As previously indicated, our ability to adapt and change in response to our environment and our personal circumstances and contexts is dependent upon neuroplastic changes in the brain. Thus, changes in the structure and function of the brain are closely tied to the process of occupational adaptation. These changes can be adaptive, leading to health and wellness, or they can be maladaptive, leading to dysfunction. Neuroplasticity begins during development and continues throughout the life span. For organizational purposes, three types of neuroplasticity will be described: developmental plasticity, synaptic plasticity, and (functional) plasticity at the modular level (Figure 3-2).

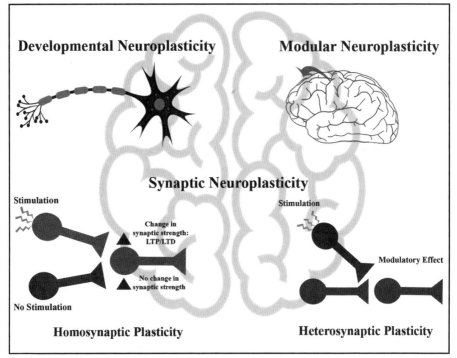

Figure 3-2. Types of adaptation. Developmental plasticity includes neurogenesis, migration, and pruning. Synaptic plasticity includes homosynaptic and heterosynaptic plasticity. Modular plasticity includes homologous area adaptation, cross-modal reassignment, map expansion, and compensatory masquerade. Abbreviations: LTD, weakening of synapse; LTP, strengthening of synapse.

Developmental Plasticity

Neuroplasticity research spans more than a century, with a significant focus on determining how neuronal structures and networks are related to how we learn. Scientists initially believed that there were limits to plasticity in that the brain could be altered early in development but that it became more hard-wired as the brain matured. Spanish neuroscientist Ramón y Cajal heavily influenced early research in the 1900s. He fostered the belief that neuroplasticity was only possible during the *critical period* in early childhood. In early development, neurons are created in overabundance. It was widely acknowledged that neurons and glial cells increased in development but that the process ceased in adolescence. Neurons go through a pruning, or *apoptosis*, in which programmed cell death occurs to control the number of neurons in babies (Wittenberg, 2009; You et al., 2005). It is now evident that pruning of superfluous networks continues throughout the lifetime but slows significantly as we age (Costandi, 2016). The neurons migrate and connect to other neurons, and there is competition to innervate a target. The typical development of the brain is influenced by the individual's genetic constitution and time-specific, sequential maturation. All of these factors must be delicately balanced in order to lay the foundation of development and learning. For example, movement in children transitions from disorganized movement patterns of infancy to more intentional and complex movement in middle childhood (Ramey & DeLuca, 2013). Rehabilitation treatment is optimal during childhood because many neurological events, such as sensory and motor development, occur by 13 years old (Cramer et al., 2011; Taub, 2004; Wittenberg, 2009).

Continued neuroplasticity into adulthood is largely attributed to experience and occurs at multiple levels within the nervous system, from changes in the type, strength, and numbers of connections between individual neurons (Sweatt, 2016) to functional changes at the representational modular level (Grafman, 2000). Each of these will be considered in turn, and although presented individually for simplicity, it should be noted that these types of plasticity are not mutually exclusive.

Synaptic Plasticity

Synaptic plasticity involves changes in the strength of connections between individual neurons and the formation of new connections between neurons that result in changes in the wiring of the brain. Cajal and fellow turn of the century neuroscientist, Eugenio Tanzi, agreed that synaptic growth is influenced by mental exercise; structural studies in the mid-1900s confirmed their assumption with the introduction of electron microscopy (Chapleau & Pozzo-Miller, 2009). Donald Hebb (1949), who is widely known as the father of neuropsychology, hypothesized that when one neuron excites another neuron repeatedly, metabolic processes take place in one or both cells that result in the strengthening of the synaptic connections between the two cells (Costandi, 2016; Jäncke, 2009; Sweatt, 2016). This process is known as *long-term potentiation* (LTP). Brain studies found that dendritic spines are affected by LTP by an increase in size, surface area, or volume. New spines can also develop along dendritic branches and in adjacent locations as a result of practice of activities. Conversely, *long-term depression* (LTD) weakens selected synapses (Costandi, 2016). LTP and LTD are examples of homosynaptic plasticity. *Homosynaptic plasticity* produces changes in communication at the synapses that were directly activated at the time of information transfer. Conversely, changes at synapse that were not active during the information transfer are called *heterosynaptic*. It is thought that heterosynaptic plasticity helps to regulate excitatory and inhibitory inputs into neuronal networks, creating homeostasis that leads to an optimal environment for learning (Chistiakova & Volgushev, 2009). The processes of homosynaptic and heterosynaptic plasticity are instrumental to our ability to learn, form memories, and adapt to our environment.

In fact, neuroscience researchers report evidence of homosynaptic and heterosynaptic plasticity at work in various areas of the brain associated with learning and memory (Sweatt, 2016). For example, there is evidence that these processes take place in the hippocampus, underlying declarative memory formation (Sweatt, 2016); the amygdala which has been implicated in associative types of learning, such as fear-conditioning (Bauer & LeDoux, 2004; Nabavi et al., 2014); the cerebellum (Hoxha, Tempia, Lippiello, & Miniaci, 2016) and basal ganglia (Wickens, 2009; Di Filippo et al., 2009), structures instrumental to motor learning (correlation-based and reward-based learning, respectively) and memory of goal directed behaviors (Dasgupta, Wörgötter, & Manoonpong, 2014), as well as various regions of the cerebral cortex (Sweatt, 2016).

Activity-dependent plasticity initiates homeostasis of individual neurons while leading to neuroadaptation based on influence from the environment (Hamaide, De Groof, & van der Linden, 2016). Experience drives the creation and elimination of synapses, and these changes are responsible for adaptive changes throughout neural networks in various regions within the brain. Adaptive changes of this sort are complex and represent forms of functional neuroplasticity at the modular level (Grafman, 2000). An examination of these more global types of plasticity is important to understanding the neural basis of occupational adaptation.

Functional Plasticity at the Modular Level

At the highest level of neuroplasticity, the network module level, Grafman (2000) has proposed four major forms of functional neuroplasticity that can be studied in humans: homologous area adaptation, cross-modal reassignment, map expansion, and compensatory masquerade. These forms of functional neuroplasticity involve cooperation between neural networks in various regions of the brain. As such, they are likely responsible for a broad range of adaptive responses that result from engagement in occupation and allow us to successfully engage in occupation.

In *homologous area adaptation*, a specific process is carried out by the homologous region in the opposite hemisphere. For example, it is well-known that the left inferior frontal gyrus (IFG) plays a dominant role in speech production, yet there is evidence that if dysfunction occurs in the left IFG, increased activity in the homologous area in the right hemisphere contributes to language function (Hartwigsen et al., 2013). This type of adaptation allows for the shifting of operations from one region of the brain to another region of the brain and is thought to occur most often during an early critical stage of development and in response to injury or disease processes (Grafman, 2000).

In *cross-modal reassignment* or *cross-modal plasticity*, an area that previously processed a particular type of sensory input now receives input from another sensory source. This type of plasticity is often the result of decreased sensory input to a cortical region. In the absence of the typical sensory input, the brain region is recruited by other sensory modalities (Glick & Sharma, 2017). Examples of cross-modal plasticity are prevalent in the literature. For example, there is evidence that cross-modal plasticity occurs due to auditory deprivation in both children and adults. Neurons in the auditory cortices of those with varying degrees of hearing loss have been shown to be responsive to both visual and somatosensory stimuli. The recruitment of the auditory cortices by other sensory modalities is likely due to the reliance on these sensory cues to aid speech perception and enhance communication abilities (Glick & Sharma, 2017).

Likewise, neuroimaging studies reveal that the visual cortices of persons with congenital or acquired blindness process tactile, auditory, and olfactory stimuli (Araneda, Renier, Rombaux, Cuevas, & De Volder, 2016; Kupers & Ptito, 2014; Lazzouni & Lepore, 2014). This type of cross-modal plasticity in persons who are blind has been associated with behavioral reports of superior abilities in processing these sensory modalities. Thus, cross-modal plasticity allows an individual to make the most efficient use of all of his or her available senses and to function and perform tasks in his or her environment despite the loss of the ability to process a particular sensory modality (Lazzouni & Lepore, 2014).

Reports of cortical reorganization involving *map expansion* are extensive and span several decades. In map expansion, a representational area carrying out a specific function expands as a result of the performance of that function or repeated exposure to a stimulus, giving meaning to the adages "we are what we do" and "practice makes perfect." This type of plasticity has been reported in various brain regions, including, but not limited to, the somatosensory cortices (Kleber et al., 2016; Mogilner et al., 1993), motor cortices (Pascual-Leone & Torres, 1993; Pascual-Leone et al., 1995; Ruffino, Papaxanthis, & Lebon, 2017), hippocampus (Maquire et al., 2000), auditory cortex (Kleber et al., 2016), and visual cortices (Mongelli et al., 2017).

Mogilner et al. (1993) used magnetoecephalography to show somatosensory reorganization in two adults who had undergone surgical separation of syndactyly. Prior to the surgery, the somatosensory maps of the fingers were shrunken and lacked the typical somatotopic organization. Post-surgery, the somatosensory representation associated with the fingers expanded over distances of 3 to 9 mm, and the cortical map was more somatotopically organized, reflecting the new functional abilities of the hand. Pascual-Leone and Torres (1993) provided further evidence of the ability of cortical regions to expand. Using transcranial magnetic stimulation (TMS), they reported that the sensorimotor cortical representation of the right index finger (reading finger) in Braille readers was expanded in comparison to their nonreading left index finger or to the right and left index fingers of control participants (Pascual-Leone & Torres, 1993).

Similarly, in a seminal study, Pascual-Leone et al. (1995) used TMS to map the motor cortices of healthy individuals as they acquired a new fine motor skill. They found enlargement of the cortical motor areas representing the long finger flexor and extensor muscles in individuals who learned to play a five-finger exercise on a piano. Participants who played the piano at will but did not practice the specific sequence also exhibited cortical map expansion; however, the expansion occurred to a lesser degree as compared to those who learned the novel sequence, suggesting that both practice and novelty are important elements that drive plasticity in the human motor system (Pascual-Leone et al., 1995). Interestingly, in a second experiment they found that simply imagining the performance of the finger piano sequence for 2 hours per day for 5 days in the absence of physical performance led to the same plastic changes in the motor system as physically practicing the skill, suggesting that mentally practicing a motor skill can promote neuroplasticity in a manner similar to physical practice of a skill (Pascual-Leone et al., 1995). A recent review of the literature confirms the notion that mentally rehearsing a physical skill leads to improved skill performance and associated cortical reorganization (Ruffino et al., 2017). This illustrates that even when we repetitively imagine engaging in occupation, the brain changes in response to that engagement.

Using structural magnetic resonance imaging (MRI), Maguire et al. (2000) reported enlargement on the posterior hippocampus and shrinkage of the anterior hippocampus in individuals with extensive navigational experience (i.e., London taxi drivers) as compared to control participants. According to the authors, the regional expansion of the posterior hippocampus was likely related to the area's role in the storage of spatial representations of the environment, providing evidence that regions of the brain change selectively in response to experience and environmental demands (Maguire et al., 2000). Similarly, experience-driven structural and functional plasticity has been observed in various regions of somatosensory, visual, and auditory cortices of both instrumental and vocal musicians (Kleber et al., 2016; Mongelli et al., 2017); in cortical and subcortical areas associated with fine motor control, procedural memory, and visual imagery in artists (Chamberlain et al., 2014); and in the primary motor cortex of individuals who were post-bilateral upper extremity amputation who developed special foot skills (e.g., recruitment of hand areas of the primary motor cortex to process motor information related to foot movements) (Yu et al., 2014). These studies underscore the notion that engagement in activity causes the brain to change and that these changes influence adaptive behavioral responses.

A final example of functional plasticity is *compensatory masquerade*. This form of plasticity involves the reorganization of preexisting neural networks. This reorganization allows the performance of a function to be carried out successfully in the absence of networks that previously supported that function. According to Grafman (2000), an example of this would be an individual who has sustained damage to neural networks underlying spatial navigation learning to navigate a route from point A to point B using explicit verbal labeling of spatial landmarks along the route. Thus, the individual uses a spared neural network to successfully complete the task in the absence of the damaged network. Grafman (2000) further indicates that this form of plasticity is an insidious process, making it difficult to study, which may explain why there are few, if any, clear experimental examples of this type of plasticity in the literature.

Although these examples depict neuroplastic changes that result from engagement in occupation and produce adaptive behavioral responses, it should be pointed out that this is not always the case. At times, plasticity can be maladaptive. For example, there is evidence that after upper limb amputation, the areas of somatosensory cortex that used to represent the hand are taken over by adjacent areas of the cortex that represent other body parts (e.g., the lip). This type of cortical expansion is associated with increased reports of phantom limb pain that interferes with function (MacIver, Lloyd, Kelly, Roberts, & Nurmikko, 2008). Furthermore, although repetitive movements are found to be beneficial to promote neuroplasticity, overuse of precise movements during occupations can be maladaptive. Furuya and Hanakawa (2016) found that repetitive, precise motor movements such as painting, writing, and performing surgery may result in a maladaptive movement disorder known as *focal-task specific dystonia* (FTSD). FTSD occurs only when the individual performs the repetitive, precise activity (e.g., a dentist drilling cavities) and does not impact other precise fine motor movements unrelated to the activity (e.g., texting on a cell phone). In addition to motor involvement, patients with FTSD are found to have sensory involvement, including spatial, temporal, and tactile deficiencies. Neural maladaptation linked to FTSD is evident in the sensory and motor cortices, basal ganglia, and cerebellum (Chen, Fremont, Arteaga-Bracho, & Khodakhah, 2014; Furuya & Hanakawa, 2016).

Whether adaptive or maladaptive, it is clear that the brain changes in response to engagement in occupation. These changes occur at the level of the synapse, resulting in the strengthening or weakening of synaptic connectivity, as well as at the representational modular level, resulting in changes in communication patterns between neural networks across multiple regions of the brain. Thus, engagement in occupation can be used to drive neuroplasticity to enhance recovery of function in the cases of injury or disease processes. The next section will review the evidence as it pertains to the brain's ability to change in response to occupational engagement after injury.

Neuroplasticity and Recovery of Function

Pathology in the brain, whether during development or as a result of disease or injury, can disrupt the functional process of plasticity (Ismail, Fatemi, & Johnston, 2016). Although there may be some spontaneous recovery, cortical reorganization takes significantly longer (Cauraugh & Summers, 2005). To complicate things, the individual may respond by developing maladaptive patterns.

It is difficult to know with certainty how neuroplastic changes in humans are behaviorally exhibited. Motor learning research over the past two decades has advanced significantly and is focused on strategies that are thought to influence neuroplasticity. Research in both children and adults suggests that engagement in goal-directed activities can promote neuroplastic changes in the brain and improved function after neurologic injury (Butler & Page, 2006; Grunt et al., 2017; Holmström et al., 2010; Sawaki et al., 2008; Wu et al., 2010), supporting the premise that occupation and the brain coeffect each other (Lohman & Royeen, 2002). For example, task-oriented training interventions such as constraint-induced movement therapy (CIMT) and bilateral repetitive task practice are known to be effective in both children with hemiplegic cerebral palsy (Schertz et al., 2016; Sterling et al., 2013) and adults post-stroke (Wolf et al., 2006; Wu et al., 2010). The core component of these interventions is the dynamic interaction between the person, task, and environment. It is important to note that research outcomes of children and adults can vary. For example, children with congenital disorders appear to differ from adults in recovery of motor function because, in general, adults have the opportunity to experience normal movement patterns or sensory feedback from those movements. There are also limitations with neuroimaging of children due to ethical considerations and decreased tolerance to undergoing MRI or other invasive techniques (Rajapakse & Kirton, 2013). Nonetheless, new technologies such as TMS and functional MRI (fMRI) have advanced our knowledge in recent years (Cauraugh & Summers, 2005). Evidence from selected intervention studies depicting behavioral changes and associated neuroplasticity are highlighted in Table 3-1 to illustrate the transactional relationship between occupational adaptation and changes in the brain.

Task-Oriented Training Interventions

Stroke and cerebral palsy are frequently cited for debilitating barriers to occupation in both adults and children. Rehabilitative interventions such as CIMT (Sawaki et al., 2008; Taub, 2004) and bimanual training using functional tasks (Wu et al., 2010) have been found to have significant impact on recovery of function.

Table 3-1

Select Intervention Studies Depicting Influence of Occupational Engagement on Neuroplasticity and Recovery of Function

Intervention	Participants	Behavioral Changes	Neuroplasticity	References
CIMT	Adults Post-stroke (n = 30; >3 and <9 months post-stroke)	Improvements in affected arm and hand function, as measured by the WMFT post-intervention and at follow-up	Map expansion in the motor cortex (hand area) ipsilesionally, as measured by TMS	Sawaki et al. (2008)
CIMT and CIMT + MP	Adults Post-stroke (n = 4; 3 to 16 months post-stroke)	Improvements in affected arm and hand function post-intervention, as measured by the WMFT for CIMT participant and 1 of the CIMT + MP participants	Cortical reorganization of bilateral motor areas, as measured by fMRI for the CIMT participant, and ipsilesional motor areas for 1 of the CIMT + MP participants	Butler and Page (2006)
CIMT & BAT	Adults Post-stroke (n = 6; >6 months post-stroke)	Improvement in motor and daily functioning, as measured by the FMA, ARAT, and MAL post-intervention	Patterns of cortical reorganization in motor areas were intervention and patient specific	Wu et al. (2010)
CIMT	Children Congenital Hemiparesis (n = 5; pre- and 1 week post-mCIMT)	Improvements with developmental disregard of impaired arm related to quality and hand use, as measured by functional assessment and grip strength	Activation in contralateral region following mCIMT, as measured by fMRI	Sutcliffe, Logan, and Fehlings (2009)
	Children Congenital Hemiparesis (n = 10; 3 weeks post)	Gains in quality and use of impaired limb, as measured by occupational therapy outcome measures	Gray matter volume increase in contralateral sensory-motor cortex and hippocampus and ipsilateral MC	Sterling et al. (2013)

(continued)

Table 3-1 (continued)

Select Intervention Studies Depicting Influence of Occupational Engagement on Neuroplasticity and Recovery of Function

Intervention	Participants	Behavioral Changes	Neuroplasticity	References
BAT	Adults Unilateral CP (n = 20) Baseline, post-HABIT and 8 to 10 weeks post	Children with most significant damage demonstrated more progress with bilateral activities but less progress with unilateral activities	Less activation on fMRI in contralesional regions during hand movement of the affected limb	Schertz et al. (2016)
MP	Adults Post-UL Amputation with PLP (n = 13)	Decrease in intensity of PLP post-intervention	Reduction in activation of hand areas of motor and sensory cortices during lip purse task, as measured by fMRI	MacIver et al. (2008)
	Children Congenital CP (n = 20)	N/A	Activation following MP tasks was decreased for participants with left-sided lesions vs right-sided lesions	Chinier et al. (2014)
MT	Adults Post-UL Amputation with Chronic PLP (n = 13)	Reduction in PLP post-intervention	Reversal of maladaptive cortical reorganization in somatosensory cortex, as measured by fMRI	Foell, Bekrater-Bodmann, Diers, and Flor (2014)
	Adults Post-stroke (n = 40; mean TPS 3.9 years; RCT	Improvements in affected arm/hand motor function, as measured by the FMA post-intervention; no changes in activity or participation measures	Shift in the balance of activation of primary motor cortex in favor of the ipsilesional hemisphere, as measured by fMRI	Michielsen et al. (2011)
	Children Hemiplegia (n = 12) and without (n = 8)	Significance found in quality of hand movement on functional testing following MT for children	Excitability found in varied regions in subjects with impairment and contralaterally in those without using TMS	Grunt et al. (2017)
	Children Hemiplegia (n = 90) RCT	Post-hoc analysis showed improvement with grip/pinch strength, UE function, accuracy, and daily performance	N/A	Bruchez et al. (2016)

(continued)

Table 3-1 (continued)

Select Intervention Studies Depicting Influence of Occupational Engagement on Neuroplasticity and Recovery of Function

Intervention	Participants	Behavioral Changes	Neuroplasticity	References
AO	Adults Post-stroke (n = 20; >6 months post-stroke) RCT	Improvement in hand dexterity, as measured by the BBT post-intervention	Activation of neural areas associated with the MSN, as measured by EEG-based brain mapping	Kuk et al. (2016)
	Children CP (n = 16)	Improvements found pre and post and significantly better vs children with grasp, spasticity, performance, and participation measures	N/A	Kim et al. (2014)
	Children Congenital Hemiparesis (n = 18)	N/A	fMRI study found recruitment in the primary motor cortex during AO of simple hand movements and consistent with adult findings	Dinomais et al. (2013)
VR training	Adults Post-stroke (n = 10; >6 months post-stroke) RCT	Improvement in arm and hand function, as measured by the FMA, BBT, and MFT	Shift in the balance of activation of primary motor cortex in favor of the ipsilesional hemisphere, as measured by fMRI	Jang et al. (2005)
	Children Case Study, 8-year-old male with hemiparesis	Improved motor performance with self-feeding, dressing, and reaching	Following VR, contralateral SMC was activated	You et al. (2005)

Abbreviations: AO, action observation; ARAT, Action Research Arm Test; BAT, bilateral arm training; BBT, Box and Blocks Test; CIMT, constraint-induced movement therapy; CP, cerebral palsy; EEG, electroencephalogram; FMA, Fugl-Meyer Assessment; fMRI, functional magnetic resonance imaging; HABIT, hand-arm bimanual intensive training; MAL, Motor Activity Log; MC, motor cortex; mCIMT, modified constraint-induced movement therapy; MFT, Manual Function Test; MNS, mirror neuron system; MP, mental practice; MT, mirror therapy; N/A, not applicable; PLP, phantom limb pain; RCT, randomized, controlled trial; SMC, sensory-motor cortex; TMS, transcranial magnetic stimulation; TPS, time post-stroke; UE, upper extremity; UL, upper limb; VR, virtual reality; WMFT, Wolf Motor Function Test.

Constraint-Induced Movement Therapy

Traditional CIMT models involve restraint of the unimpaired upper limb coupled with repetitive task training of the impaired upper limb during functionally based activities (e.g., eating, writing, folding laundry) and the behavioral conditioning principle of *shaping*, which involves the presentation of repetitive activities with immediate rewards (e.g., verbal praise, food, gestures) and a progressive increase in difficulty. Repetitive tasks are highly structured by nature but can also be challenging and motivating (Ramey & DeLuca, 2013). According to Taub (2004), upper extremity activities that involve repeated practice of functional movements promote growth in the contralateral cortical area and recruit new areas in ipsilateral regions of the brain. Thus, activity-dependent plasticity occurs when the affected arm is used with repeated and sustained practice of task-related movements. The traditional training is provided for 6 hours a day for 21 consecutive days (Taub, 2004; Uswatte & Taub, 2005) or 6 hours for 2 weeks (Sawaki et al., 2008). However, modified versions of CIMT that reduce the restraint time of the unimpaired limb and/or reduce the intensive training or distribute the training over longer periods of time are also effective at improving function (Case-Smith, DeLuca, Stevenson, & Ramey, 2012; Shi, Tian, Yang, & Zhao, 2011).

In addition to the positive behavioral changes attributed to CIMT, cortical reorganization has been reported post-training in both children (Sterling et al., 2013; Sutcliff, Logan, & Fehlings, 2009) and adults (Butler & Page, 2006; Sawaki et al., 2008). In a pediatric study on children with congenital hemiplegia, Sutcliffe et al. (2009) found fMRI changes in activation of the contralesional side and improved use and quality of movement following CIMT. Similarly, Sterling et al. (2013) found structural changes in gray matter of the sensory-motor cortex (SMC), hippocampus, and ipsilateral motor cortex (MC), along with improvement in hand use and quality in children with hemiparesis following CIMT. Using TMS to map the motor cortex of adult stroke survivors in the subacute phase of recovery who had undergone CIMT training, Sawaki et al. (2008) reported map expansion in the hand area of the ipsilesional motor cortex that was correlated with improved lifting force and grip strength in the paretic hand. Butler and Page (2006) reported that stroke patients participating in a 2-week CIMT intervention or CIMT combined with mental practice intervention improved motor function of the involved upper extremity that was associated with cortical reorganization of the involved hemisphere as measured by fMRI.

Bilateral Training

Whereas CIMT focuses on engagement in occupation using only the affected limb, bimanual training involves repetitive use of both the impaired and nonimpaired hand and is commonly used to treat pediatric and adult hemiplegia. It is postulated that neural activation occurs during the use of the unaffected arm and bilateral limb practice may aid in the recovery of damaged networks (Cauraugh & Summers, 2005). Wu et al. (2010) reported improved motor and daily functioning in chronic stroke survivors after they received either a distributed form of CIMT (dCIMT) or intensive bilateral arm training (BAT) during functional tasks. Interestingly, these improvements were associated with various patterns of cortical reorganization that were participant and intervention specific, illustrating that neuroplastic changes after stroke are the result of dynamic interactions between the person and the task training. For example, during bilateral elbow movements, the group that received BAT showed increased activation in the cerebellum bilaterally, whereas the group receiving dCIMT showed decreased activation patterns. Also, participants exhibiting the greatest functional changes post-intervention had large increases in activation of the ipsilesional MC during affected hand movements, regardless of the training regime. Schertz et al. (2016) conducted a fMRI with children with unilateral cerebral palsy who participated in an intensive BAT program. Neuroactivation was strongly correlated with improvements of the affected limb using bilateral activity, but showed a negative correlation between neuroactivation and unilateral activity with only the affected arm. These studies illustrate that, regardless of age, as individuals attempt to engage in activity despite illness or injury, the brain changes in response to those attempts. Rehabilitation research suggests that engagement in novel activities also plays an important role in changing the brain.

Engagement in Novel Activities

Engagement in novel activities, such as task training using virtual reality (VR) or combining task training with cognitive strategies such as mental practice (imagined engagement in occupation), action observation (watching another person engaging in occupation with the intention of imitating that engagement), or mirror therapy (watching the mirror reflection of oneself engaged in task performance), may promote recovery of function in both children (Bruchez et al,. 2016; Kim, Kim, & Ko, 2014) and adults (Butler & Page, 2006; MacIver et al., 2008; Michielsen et al., 2011). Research that examines neuroimaging and novel activities is presented here. It must be noted that pediatric studies that encompass both neuroimaging and novel activities are relatively nonexistent; therefore, the pediatric studies presented may entail an example of one or the other.

Mental Practice

During *mental practice*, an individual imagines engaging in an activity with the purpose of enhancing performance of that activity. Evidence suggests that this imagined effort activates areas of the brain that are similar to those that are active during actual engagement of the activity (Butler & Page, 2006). As indicated earlier, Butler and Page (2006) found evidence that this type of training, when combined with CIMT, improves function in stroke survivors and is associated with changes in the organization of the damaged motor cortex. Mental practice has also been reported to be effective at reversing the maladaptive motor and somatosensory cortical reorganization associated with phantom limb pain (MacIver et al., 2008). The reversal of this maladaptive cortical reorganization is correlated with decreases in the intensity of constant phantom limb pain after upper limb amputation (MacIver et al., 2008). In a pediatric study using fMRI, Chinier et al. (2014) discovered that when children with unilateral cerebral palsy participate in motor imagery of simple hand movements, bilateral activation in the frontal lobe occurs. Motor imagery was more effective with children with right brain lesions than those with left brain lesions. In addition to motor imagery, mirror therapy demonstrates a significant linkage between neuroplasticity and clinical task performance.

Mirror Therapy

Mirror therapy is a treatment method that has been successfully used to reduce phantom limb pain after upper limb amputation (Foell et al., 2014) and to improve motor performance in stroke survivors (Thieme, Mehrholz, Pohl, Behrens, & Dohle, 2012) and children with cerebral palsy (Bruchez et al., 2016; Grunt et al., 2017). During mirror therapy, a person engages in a task using one extremity while viewing the mirror reflection of that extremity superimposed over the unseen extremity. This mirror visual feedback (MVF) creates a visual illusion that both extremities are simultaneously engaged in task performance. A recent review of the literature investigating the effects of MVF on the brain suggest this type of feedback activates higher-order neural areas associated with attention and action monitoring, as well as areas associated with the mirror neuron system (i.e., superior temporal gyrus and premotor cortex) and the motor network (i.e., primary motor cortices). In addition, it appears that MVF promotes cortical reorganization associated with adaptive behavioral responses that support recovery of function post-injury (Deconinck et al., 2015).

For example, Foell et al. (2014) reported that a daily mirror training program provided significantly reduced phantom limb pain over 4 weeks in a cohort of participants with chronic phantom limb pain following an upper extremity amputation. This reduction in pain was associated with a reversal of maladaptive somatosensory cortical reorganization (e.g., reduction of activity in the inferior parietal cortex in the hemisphere affected by the amputation, such that the representational areas in somatosensory cortex of both hemispheres were more similar).

Michielsen et al. (2011) reported cortical reorganization (i.e., shift in activation balance within primary motor cortex toward the ipsilesional hemisphere) following a 6-week mirror therapy program in chronic stroke survivors. This cortical reorganization was associated with improved motor function in the involved arm and hand post-intervention (Michielsen et al., 2011). In a TMS study, Grunt et al. (2017) found that children with hemiplegia showed increased excitability that was associated with improved hand quality of movement following mirror therapy. Another cognitive strategy used to improve motor skill learning that shows promise in cortical reorganization involves action observation.

Action Observation

During *action observation*, one person watches another person engaged in an activity with the intention of physically performing the activity themselves. Observation of another in action activates areas associated with the mirror neuron system (i.e., premotor cortex, inferior frontal gyrus, and posterior parietal lobe). This action execution–matching system allows us to understand other's actions as well as learn from them. Evidence suggests that this system can be tapped to promote cortical reorganization and recovery of function post-injury (Buccino, 2014). For example, a recent study investigating the effects of action observation on motor recovery of the involved hand post-stroke reported improved dexterity and associated changes in cortical activation patterns in brain areas associated with the mirror neuron system, as measured by electroencephalogram-based brain mapping (Kuk, Kim, Oh, & Hwang, 2016). Dinomais et al. (2013) conducted a pediatric fMRI study to identify neuroactivation following action observation of simple hand movement and found that the bilateral motor cortices and cerebellum were activated regardless of severity of impairment. In another clinical study, action observation was found to significantly improve occupational therapy measures of hand function, performance, and participation (Kim et al., 2014). Changes in neuroactivation and function/participation are apparent across the developmental spectrum through the use of task-oriented cognitive activities. Likewise, VR has been found to show significance with both neural changes and performance in activities.

Virtual Reality

One emerging area of rehabilitation is VR, which consists of computer technology that provides sensory-rich experiences similar to real-life activities. VR supports motor learning theory as the patient receives continuous performance feedback from information presented on the computer screen (Snider, Majnemer, & Darsaklis, 2010). fMRI studies have shown cortical activation of the affected elbow was reorganized from bilateral SMC and from ipsilateral supplementary motor area (SMA) (pre) to contralateral SMC (post). This may suggest that VR rehabilitation improves neuroplasticity, which can generate synaptic potentiation and motor performance by imitation (You et al., 2005). VR has other advantages, including: the ability to easily grade the complexity of the therapeutic activity, allowing the child to explore increasingly complex environments, and being motivational to the child (Reid, 2004; Snider et al., 2010). Reid (2004) states that VR promotes active engagement of occupation through neuroplastic activity-dependent treatment appropriate for children with hemiplegia.

Similarly, VR training has been successfully applied to adults post-stroke to improve arm and hand function. Jang et al. (2005) found that a task-oriented training program using VR provided for 60 minutes per day, 5 times per week, for 4 weeks, improved arm and hand function as measured by the Fugl-Meyer Motor Assessment (FMA), Box and Blocks Test (BBT), and Manual Function Test (MFT), above a control condition. Furthermore, improved arm and hand function were associated with cortical activation shifts toward the affected motor cortex during affected arm movements as measured by fMRI (Jang et al., 2005). Based on the studies explored, there appears to be a confluence of adult and pediatric research that draws a distinct connection between task-oriented training novel activity and neuroplasticity.

The following case study about Jacob depicts his participation in a combination of task-oriented interventions (CIMT and bilateral training) along with engagement in novel activities via the use of VR.

CASE STUDY: JACOB Jacob is a 6-year-old boy with right-side congenital hemiplegia. He participated in a 4-week CIMT summer day camp. A variety of assessments were conducted before, after, and 6 months post-camp, including the impairment focused assessments of hand function and assessments of occupational participation. The first 3 weeks of intervention were focused on engagement in occupation, with activities using only the left hand while the right arm was in a removable cast. Jacob and his family agreed to follow through with typical activities at home while wearing the cast. Camp activities consisted of structured craft, music, recreation, and daily living activities and novel and repetitive activities using a VR system. The therapist, Mary, designed the activities and facilitated the camp in order to provide enough challenge but also made frequent adjustments to minimize frustration. Jacob chose a variety of ongoing activities (e.g., bocce ball vs Frisbee golf, the type of game on the VR system, etc.) throughout camp to ensure continuous engagement. The fourth week of intervention involved bilateral training, with engagement in occupations at camp and at home.

At times during the camp, Jacob became frustrated because his right hand would not work as he wanted. This would manifest as him crying or shouting at his hand during group. He and Mary talked through each task that was causing the frustration as it occurred. For example, with a shoe-tying activity, Mary broke down the steps and began with the backward chaining technique (all steps performed by Mary except the last one). They also decided that Jacob would teach her to tie her shoe with one hand. To reinforce at home, Mary showed him an online video that demonstrated adaptive shoe tying and provided the web link to his mother.

Following camp, fMRI studies showed more activation in the primary sensorimotor cortex of the affected hemisphere. Jacob said he was excited because he could use his right hand better and faster while playing Minecraft and grabbing flags during flag football. His mother reported that he was less frustrated with simple things like opening drinks, cutting meat, and tying his shoes. Overall, participation in the summer camp showed not only neuroplastic changes but also improvement in Jacob's efficiency, efficacy, and satisfaction in his occupational performance.

ADVANCING THE EVIDENCE OF OCCUPATIONAL ADAPTATION

Research on the relationship between neuroplasticity and the adaptive capacity during participation in occupation is admittedly sparse. A primary reason is directly related to impracticality of neuroimaging while performing real-life activities. Although not explicitly stated in much of the research, we found substantial evidence that may suggest that neuroplasticity and occupational adaptation are processes that are dynamically interconnected. Occupational therapists attempt to facilitate occupational adaptation in our clients through the careful design of activities following a life-changing event. We provide guidance for the client to find novel ways of doing occupations to either create a new sense of self or overcome contextual barriers. From a neuroplasticity perspective, a crucial element to the adaptive process is to remap the brain to encourage the client's optimal function and, ultimately, participation in occupations in new and different ways following disease or injury.

SUMMARY AND IMPLICATIONS

- Simple and complex forms of behavioral adaptation rely on unique patterns of neuronal communication.
- Evidence suggests that neuroplasticity occurs in response to human development, engagement in activities, and transaction with the environment and as a consequence of disease or injury.
- Combined neuroimaging and behavioral studies suggest that engagement in activity post-injury promotes adaptive changes in the brain and improves function.
- Although the evidence suggests that the brain and occupation coeffect each other, further studies that specifically measure occupational adaptation and associated neuroplastic changes are needed.

REFERENCES

Araneda, R., Renier, L. A., Rombaux, P., Cuevas, I., & De Volder, A. G. (2016). Cortical plasticity and olfactory function in early blindness. *Frontiers in Systems Neuroscience, 10*, 75. doi:10.3389/fnsys.2016.00075

Bauer, E. P., & LeDoux, J. E. (2004). Heterosynaptic long-term potentiation of inhibitory interneurons in the lateral amygdala. *Journal of Neuroscience, 24*, 9507-9512. doi:10.1523/jneurosci.3567-04.2004

Bruchez, R., Jequier Gygax, M., Roches, S., Fluss, J., Jacquier, D., Balleni, P., … Newman, C. J. (2016). Mirror therapy in children with hemiparesis: A randomized observer-blinded trial. *Developmental Medicine and Child Neurology, 58*(9), 970-978. doi:10.111/dmcn.13117

Buccino, G. (2014). Action observation treatment: a novel tool in neurorehabilitation. *Philosophical Transactions of the Royal Society, 369*, 20130185. doi:10.1098/rstb.2013.0185

Butler, A. J., & Page, S. J. (2006). Mental practice with motor imagery: evidence for motor recovery and cortical reorganization. *Archives of Physical Medicine and Rehabilitation, 87*(12), S2-S11. doi:10.1016/j.apmr.2006.08.326

Byrne, J. H. (n.d.). Introduction to neurons and neuronal networks. In J. H. Byrne (Ed.), *Neuroscience online: An electronic textbook for the neurosciences*. Retrieved from https://www.youtube.com/watch?v=nlSL7Qg7-Po

Case-Smith, J., DeLuca, S. C., Stevenson, R., & Ramey, S. L. (2012). Multicenter randomized controlled trial of pediatric constraint-induced movement therapy: 6 month follow-up. *American Journal of Occupational Therapy, 66*(1), 15-23.

Cauraugh, J. H., & Summers, J. J. (2005). Neural plasticity and bilateral movements: A rehabilitation approach for chronic stroke. *Progress in Neurobiology, 75*(5), 309-320.

Chamberlain, R., McManus, I. C., Brunswick, N., Rankin, Q., Riley, H., & Kanai, R. (2014). Drawing on the right side of the brain: a voxel-based morphometry analysis of observational drawing. *Neuroimage, 96*, 167-173.

Chapleau, C. A., & Pozzo-Miller, L. (2009). Activity-dependent structural plasticity of dendritic spines. In J. Byrne (Ed.), *Concise learning and memory: The editor's selection.* (pp. 281-305). Oxford, England: Elsevier.

Chen, C. H., Fremont, R., Arteaga-Bracho, E. E., & Khodakhah, K. (2014). Short latency cerebellar modulation of the basal ganglia. *Nature Neuroscience, 17*, 1767-1775. doi:10.1038/nn.3868

Chinier, E., N'Guyen, S., Lignon, G., Ter Minassian, A., Richard, I., & Dinomais, M. (2014) Effect of motor imagery in children with unilateral cerebral palsy: fMRI study. *Public Library of Science ONE, 9*(4), e93378. doi:10.1371/journal.pone.0093378

Chistiakova, M., & Volgushev, M. (2009). Heterosynaptic plasticity in the neocortex. *Experimental Brain Research, 199*(3-4), 377-390.

Costandi, M. (2016). *Neuroplasticity.* Cambridge, MA: MIT Press.

Cramer, S. C., Sur, M., Dobkin, B. H., O'Brien, C., Sanger, T. D., Trojanowski, J. Q., … Vinogradov, S. (2011). Harnessing neuroplasticity for clinical applications. *Brain, 134*, 1591-1609.

Dasgupta, S., Wörgötter, F., & Manoonpong, P. (2014). Neuromodulatory adaptive combination of correlation-based learning in cerebellum and reward-based learning in basal ganglia for goal-directed behavioral control. *Front Neural Circuits, 8*, 216. doi:10.3389/fncir.2014.00126

Deconinck, F. J., Smorenburg, A. R., Benham, A., Ledebt, A., Feltham, M. G., Savelsbergh, G. J. (2015). Reflections on mirror therapy: a systematic review of the effect of mirror visual feedback on the brain. *Neurorehabilitation and Neural Repair, 29*(4), 349-361. doi:10.1177/1545968314546134

Di Filippo, M., Picconi, B., Tantucci, M., Ghiglieri, V., Bagetta, V., Sgobio C., … Calabresi, P. (2009). Short-term and long-term plasticity at corticostriatial synapses: implications for learning and memory. *Behavioural Brain Research, 199*(1), 108-118. doi:10.1016/j.bbr.2008.09.025

Dinomais, M., Lignon, G., Chinier, E., Richard, I., Ter Minassian, A., & Tich, S. N. (2013). Effect of observation of simple hand movement on brain activations in patients with unilateral cerebral palsy: An fMRI study. *Research in Developmental Disabilities, 34*(6), 1928-1937. doi:10.1016/j.ridd.2013.03.020

Foell, J., Bekrater-Bodmann, R., Diers, M., & Flor, H. (2014). Mirror therapy for phantom limb pain: brain changes and the role of body representation. *European Journal of Pain, 18*(5), 729-739. doi:10.1002/j.1532-2149.2013.00433.x

Furuya, S., & Hanakawa, T. (2016). The curse of motor expertise: Use-dependent focal dystonia as a manifestation of maladaptive changes in body representation. *Neuroscience Research, 104*, 112-119. doi:10.1016/j.neures.2015.12.001

Glick, H., & Sharma, A. (2017). Cross-modal plasticity in developmental and age-related hearing loss: clinical implications. *Hearing Research, 343*, 191-201. doi:10.1016/j.heares.2016.08.012

Grafman, J. (2000). Conceptualizing functional neuroplasticity. *Journal of Communication Disorders, 33*(4), 345-356.

Grajo, L. (2017). Occupational adaptation. In J. Hinojosa, P. Kramer, & C. Royeen (Eds.), *Perspectives on human occupation: Theories underlying practice* (2nd ed., pp. 287-311). Philadelphia, PA: F.A. Davis.

Grunt, S., Newman, C. J., Saxer, S., Steinlin, M., Weisstanner, C., & Kaelin-Lang, A. (2017). The mirror illusion increases motor cortex excitability in children with and without hemiparesis. *Neurorehabilitation & Neural Repair, 31*(3), 280-289. doi:10.1177/1545968316680483

Hamaide, J., De Groof, G., & van der Linden, A. (2016). Neuroplasticity and MRI: A perfect match. *NeuroImage, 131*, 13-28. doi:10.1016/j.neuroimage.2015.08.005

Hartwigsen, G., Saur, D., Price, C. J., Ulmer, S., Baumgaertner, A., & Siebner, H. R. (2013). Perturbation of the left inferior frontal gyrus triggers adaptive plasticity in the right homologous area during speech production. *Proceedings of the National Academy of Sciences of the United States of America, 110*(41), 16402-16407. doi:10.1073/pnas.1310190110

Hebb, D. O. (1949). *The organization of behavior: A neuropsychological theory.* Oxford, England: Wiley.

Holmström, L., Vollmer, B., Tedroff, K., Islam, M., Persson, J. K., Kits, A., … Eliasson, A. (2010). Hand function in relation to brain lesions and corticomotor projection pattern in children with unilateral cerebral palsy. *Developmental Medicine & Child Neurology, 52*(2), 145-152.

Hoxha, E., Tempia, F., Lippiello, P., & Miniaci, M. C. (2016). Modulation, plasticity, and pathophysiology of the parallel fiber-Purkinje cell synapse. *Frontiers in Synaptic Neuroscience, 8*, 35. doi:10.3389/fnsyn.2016.00035

Ismail, F. Y., Fatemi, A., & Johnston, M. V. (2016). Cerebral plasticity: Windows of opportunity developing brain. *European Journal of Paediatric Neurology, 21*(1), 23-48. doi:10.1016/j.ejpn.2016.07.007

Jäncke, L. (2009). The plastic human brain. *Restorative Neurology and Neuroscience, 27*(5), 521-538. doi:10.3233/RNN-2009-0519

Jang, S. H., You, S. H., Hallet, M., Cho, Y. W., Park, C. M., Cho, S. H., … Kim, T. (2005). Cortical reorganization and associated functional motor recovery after virtual reality in patients with chronic stroke: an experimenter-blind preliminary study. *Archives of Physical Medicine and Rehabilitation, 86*(11), 2218-2223. doi:10.1016/j.apmr.2005.04.015

Kim, J. Y., Kim, J. M., & Ko, E. Y. (2014). The effect of the action observation physical training on the upper extremity function in children with cerebral palsy. *Journal of Exercise Rehabilitation, 10*(3), 176-183. doi:10.12965/jer.140114

Kleber, B., Veit, R., Moll, C. V., Gaser, C., Birbaumer, N., & Lotze, M. (2016). Voxel-based morphometry in opera singers: increased gray-matter volume in right somatosensory and auditory cortices. *NeuroImage, 133,* 477-483.

Kuk, E. J., Kim, J. M., Oh, D. W., & Hwang, H. J. (2016). Effects of action observation therapy on hand dexterity and EEG-based cortical activation patterns in patients with post-stroke hemiparesis. *Topics in Stroke Rehabilitation, 23*(5), 318-325. doi:10.1080/10749357.2016.1157972

Kupers. 'R., & Ptito, M. (2014). Compensatory plasticity and cross-modal reorganization following early visual deprivation. *Neuroscience and Biobehavioral Reviews, 41,* 36-52.

Lazzouni, L., & Lepore, F. (2014). Compensatory plasticity: Time matters. *Frontiers in Human Neuroscience, 8,* 340. doi:10.3389/fnhum.2014.00340

Lohman, H., & Royeen, C. (2002). Posttraumatic stress disorder and traumatic hand injuries: A neuro-occupational view. *American Journal of Occupational Therapy, 56*(5), 527-537.

MacIver, K., Lloyd, D. M., Kelly, S., Roberts, N., & Nurmikko. T. (2008). Phantom limb pain, cortical reorganization and the therapeutic effect of mental imagery. *Brain, 131*(Pt. 8), 2181-2191.

Maguire, E. A., Gadian, D. G., Johnsrude, I. S., Good, C. D., Ashburner, J., Frackowiak, R. S., & Frith, C. D. (2000). Navigation-related structural change in the hippocampi of taxi drivers. *Proceedings of the National Academy of Sciences of the United States of America, 97*(8), 4398-4403.

Michielsen M. E., Selles R. W., van der Geest J. N., Eckhardt, M., Yavuzer, G., Stam, H. J., ... Bussmann, J. B. (2011). Motor recovery and cortical reorganization after mirror therapy in chronic stroke patients: a phase II randomized controlled trial. *Neurorehabilitation and Neural Repair, 25*(3), 223-233. doi:10.1177/1545968310385127

Mogilner, A., Grossman, J. A., Ribary, U., Joliot, M., Volkmann, J., Rapaport, D., ... Llinás, R. R. (1993). Somatosensory cortical plasticity in adult humans revealed by magnetoencephalography. *Proceedings of the National Academy of Sciences of the United States of America, 90*(8), 3593-3597.

Mongelli, V., Dehaene, S., Vinckier, F., Peretz, I., Bartolomeo, P., & Cohen, L. (2017). Music and words in the visual cortex: The impact of musical expertise. *Cortex, 86,* 260-274. doi:10.1016/j.cortex.2016.05.016

Nabavi, S., Fox, R., Proulx, C. D., Lin, J. Y., Tsien, R. Y., & Malinow, R. (2014). Engineering a memory with LTD and LTP. *Nature, 511*(7509), 348-352. doi:10.1038/nature13294

Pascual-Leone, A., Nguyet, D., Cohen, L. G., Brasil-Neto, J. P., Cammarota, A., & Hallett, M. (1995). Modulation of muscle responses evoked by transcranial magnetic stimulation during the acquisition of new fine motor skills. *Journal of Neurophysiology, 74*(3), 1037-1045.

Pascual-Leone, A., & Torres, F. (1993). Plasticity of the sensorimotor cortex representation of the reading finger in Braille readers. *Brain, 116*(Pt. 1), 39-52.

Rajapakse, T., & Kirton, A. (2013). Non-invasive brain stimulation in children: Applications and future directions. *Translational Neuroscience, 4*(2). doi:10.2478/s13380-013-0116-3

Ramey, S. L., & DeLuca, S. C. (2013). Pediatric CIMT: History and definition. In S. L. Ramey, P. Coker-Bolt, & S. C. DeLuca (Eds.), *Handbook of pediatric constraint induced movement therapy (CIMT): A guide for occupational therapy and health care clinicians, researchers and educators* (pp. 3-18). Bethesda, MD: AOTA Press.

Reid, D. (2004). Virtual reality and the person-environment experience. *CyberPsychology & Behavior, 5*(6), 559-564. doi:10.1089/109493102321018204

Ruffino, C., Papaxanthis, C., & Lebon, F. (2017). Neural plasticity during motor learning and motor imagery practice: Review and perspectives. *Neuroscience, 341,* 61-78. doi:10.1016/j.neuroscience.2016.11.023

Sawaki, L., Butler, A. J., Leng, X., Wassenaar, P. A., Mohammad, Y. M., Blanton, S., ... Wittenberg, G. F. (2008). Constraint-induced movement therapy resulted in increased motor map area in subjects 3 to 9 months post-stroke. *Neurorehabilitation and Neural Repair, 22*(5), 505-513. doi:10.1177/1545968308317531

Schertz, M., Shiran, S. I., Myers, V., Weinstein, M., Fattal-Valevski, A., Artzi, M., ... Green, D. (2016). Imaging predictors of improvement from a motor learning based intervention for children with unilateral cerebral palsy. *Neurorehabilitation and Neural Repair, 30*(7), 647-660. doi:10.1177/1545968315613446

Shi, Y. X., Tian, J. H., Yang, K. H., Zhao, Y. (2011). Modified constraint-induced movement therapy versus traditional rehabilitation in patients with upper extremity dysfunction after stroke: A systematic review and meta-analysis. *Archives of Physical Medicine and Rehabilitation, 92*(6), 972-982.

Snider, L., Majnemer, A., & Darsaklis, V. (2010). Virtual reality as a therapeutic modality for children with cerebral palsy. *Developmental Neurorehabilitation, 13*(2), 120-128. doi:10.3109/17518420903357753

Sterling, C., Taub, E., Davis, D., Rickards, T., Gauthier, L. V., Griffin, A., & Uswatte, G. (2013). Structural neuroplastic change after constraint-induced movement therapy in children with cerebral palsy. *Pediatrics, 131*(5), e1664-e1669. doi:10.1542/peds.2012-2051

Sutcliffe, T. L., Logan, W. J., & Fehlings, D. L. (2009). Pediatric constraint-induced movement therapy is associated with increased contralateral cortical activity on functional magnetic resonance imaging. *Journal of Child Neurology, 24*(10), 1230-1235. doi:10.1177/0883073809341268

Sweatt, J. D. (2016). Neural plasticity and behavior—Sixty years of conceptual advances. *Journal of Neurochemistry, 139*(Suppl. 2), 179-199. doi:10.1111/jnc.13580

Taub, E. (2004). Harnessing brain plasticity through behavioral techniques to produce new treatments in neurorehabilitation. *American Psychologist, 59*(8), 692-704. doi:10.1037/0003-066X.59.8.692

Thieme, H., Mehrholz, J., Pohl, M., Behrens, J., & Dohle, C. (2012). Mirror therapy for improving motor function after stroke. *Cochrane Database Syst Rev, 14*(3), CD008449.

Uswatte, G., & Taub, E. (2005). Implications of the learned nonuse formulation for measuring rehabilitation outcomes: Lessons from constraint-induced movement therapy. *Rehabilitation Psychology, 50,* 34-42. doi:10.1037/0090-5550.50.1.34

Wickens, J. R. (2009). Synaptic plasticity in the basal ganglia. *Behavioural Brain Research, 199*(1), 119-128. doi:10.1016/j.bbr.2008.10.030

Wittenberg, G. F. (2009). Neural plasticity and treatment across the lifespan for motor deficits in cerebral palsy. *Developmental Medicine and Child Neurology, 51*(Suppl. 4), 130-133. doi:10.1111/j.1469-8749.2009.03425.x

Wu, C., Hsieh, Y., Lin, K., Chuang, L., Chang, Y., Liu, H., … Wai, Y. (2010). Brain reorganization after bilateral arm training and distributed constraint-induced therapy in stroke patients: A preliminary functional magnetic resonance imaging study. *Chang Gung Medical Journal, 33*(6), 628-638. Retrieved from http://memo.cgu.edu.tw/cgmj/3306/330605.pdf

Wolf, S. L., Winstein, C. J., Miller, J. P., Taub, E., Uswatte, G., Morris D., … EXCITE Investigators. (2006). Effect of constraint-induced movement therapy on upper extremity function 3 to 9 months after stroke: the EXCITE randomized clinical trial. *JAMA: Journal of the American Medical Association, 296*(17), 2095-2104.

You, S. H., Jang, S. H., Kim, Y. H., Kwon, Y. H., Barrow, I., & Hallett, M. (2005). Cortical reorganization induced by virtual reality therapy in a child with hemiparetic cerebral palsy. *Developmental Medicine and Child Neurology, 47*(9), 628-635.

Yu, X. J., He, H. J., Zhang, Q. W., Zhao, F., Zee, C. S., Zhang, S. Z., & Gong, X. Y. (2014). Somatotopic reorganization of hand representation in bilateral arm amputees with or without special foot movement skill. *Brain Research, 1546,* 9-17. doi:10.1016/j.brainres.2013.12.025

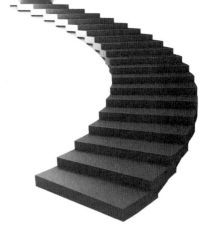

4

Neural Basis of Adaptation
Motivation, Intention, Resilience, and Goal-Directed Behaviors

Katherine Dimitropoulou, PhD, OTR and
Mary Frances Baxter, PhD, OT, FAOTA

OVERVIEW In this chapter, occupational adaptation is defined as a neurobiological process guided by cognitive and emotional systems to support growth, occupational engagement, and health. Goal-directed behavior and intention, motivation, and resilience critically contribute to this process. As described in Chapter 3, early experiences in conjunction with genetic and epigenetic factors shape neural processes underlying occupational adaptation throughout the life span. Changes in health and well-being as a result of trauma or prolonged exposure to stressors (biological or psychological) critically affect neural networks and their adaptability. In return, neuroplastic changes reflect a person's resources for occupational adaptation and his or her ability to cope with adversity or trauma, thus influencing the recovery process.

Grajo LC, Boisselle AK, eds.
Adaptation Through Occupation:
Multidimensional Perspectives (pp 59-80).
© 2019 SLACK Incorporated.

CHAPTER OBJECTIVES By the end of this chapter, the reader will be able to:

- Describe the structure and function of major cognitive and emotional networks related to motivation, intention, goal-directed behavior, and resilience that are critical for the process of adaptation.
- Describe neuroplasticity and behavioral indicators of health and recovery that are indicative of occupational adaptation.
- Describe evidence that illustrates the interplay between occupational engagement and cognitive/emotional neural mechanisms of adaptation.

QUESTIONS FOR DISCUSSION AND REFLECTION As the reader explores this chapter, let the following questions guide discussion and reflection:

- How will knowledge of neural structures and mechanisms aid my understanding of motivation, intentional and goal-directed behaviors, and resilience as they relate to the adaptation process of humans?
- How can I articulate occupational adaptation in practice, teaching, and/or research using my understanding of the processes of motivation, intentionality, and resilience?

INTRODUCTION

Between stimulus and response there is a space. In that space is our power to choose our response. In our response lies our growth and our freedom.

—Viktor Frankl, 1959

Dr. Frankl was a neurologist, psychiatrist, and a Holocaust survivor whose words capture the many possibilities of the adaptation process. He depicts the essence that one has the freedom and the potential to grow from challenging life experiences, a process that heavily depends on how people choose to interpret and explain these experiences to inform further actions, occupations, and their lifestyle (Fine, 1991). *Occupational adaptation* is the person's ability to respond positively to occupational changes and challenges that affect engagement, participation, and performance in occupations and the fulfillment of occupational roles (Grajo, 2017; Schkade & McClung, 2001; Schkade & Schultz, 1992; Schultz & Schkade, 1992).

Complex neurobiological systems of intention and goal-directed action, motivation, and resilience dynamically regulate the process of occupational adaptation. Neural plasticity and experience guide occupational adaptation in health and wellness conditions, as well as during prolonged exposure to stress (biological or psychological) and trauma (Grajo, 2017). Neuroplastic changes influence occupational adaptation and the ability to cope with occupational demands.

The interplay between neural cognitive and emotional networks regulates the process of adaptation. A variety of anatomic brain structures and their functional connectivity underlie behavioral responses that can be *adaptive* (promote occupational engagement, learning, growth, and health) vs *maladaptive* (promote stagnation, occupational deprivation, and harm). Major brain regions involved in this process are the prefrontal cortex, cingulate cortex, basal ganglia, and midbrain, with significant connections to other cortical (i.e., sensory and motor primary and association areas) and subcortical regions (i.e., amygdala, hippocampus, and endocrine systems) (Hare, Camerer, & Rangel, 2009; Kahnt et al., 2009; Kandel, Schwartz, Jessell, Siegelbaum, & Hudspeth, 2013; Leung & Balleine, 2013). Neurochemical connections between these systems facilitate prediction, identification, and memory of a person's actions (Belujon & Grace, 2015; Cao et al., 2010; Kandel et al., 2013). Development, lifestyle changes, and health and wellness challenges impose a need for an adaptive process to accommodate the changing bodies, tasks, and environments. Although the purpose of this chapter is not to provide an extensive account of neuroanatomical structures and their function, the following brief overview is important to provide contextual reference (see Chapter 3 for other descriptions of neural structures related to adaptation). We then describe the process of adaptation in these systems under different change or challenge conditions.

INTENT, GOAL-DIRECTED ACTION, MOTIVATION, AND RESILIENCE: OVERVIEW OF NEURONAL CIRCUITS

Neural Structures and Their Functional Connections

When engaging in occupations, a multitude of possibilities for action (behavioral and motor) are available for the individual. Recent theoretical frameworks about the brain suggest that task engagement entails two basic processes: deciding what to do and how to do it (Cisek & Kalaska, 2010). These two processes occur simultaneously and, in an integrated way, appropriate to support adaptive behavior in response to changing task demands (Cisek, 2007). In this perspective, actions comprise *intent* (selection of what the action will be) and the *specifications* (specify the spatiotemporal parameters of action) needed to match the task and environmental demands (Cisek & Kalaska, 2010). Evaluation of the anticipated value and the rewards from the action (*motivation*) significantly contribute to action selections. Selection of actions includes identification of actions and behaviors to support health promotion and wellness, or actions that can hinder the person's well-being. Resilience signifies choices that lead toward health and wellness, and it is critical for individual growth and recovery from trauma and adversity (Fine, 1991; Kandel et al., 2013).

Intentionality, goal-directed behaviors, motivation, and resilience entail a wide array of neural structures. The primary sensory areas (e.g., visual, somatosensory, auditory, olfactory) and secondary sensory association areas such as the medial and inferior parietal lobes (where information from multiple senses are integrated) detect stimuli that warrant action and the initiation of possible actions (Balleine & O'Doherty, 2010; Kandel et al., 2013). The prefrontal cortex, basal ganglia, amygdala, hippocampus, anterior cingulate cortex, and supplementary motor area activate according to the nature of the signal and regulatory state of the individual. This process narrows the possible eligible actions (via a selection/pruning process described in Chapter 3) to facilitate the individual's

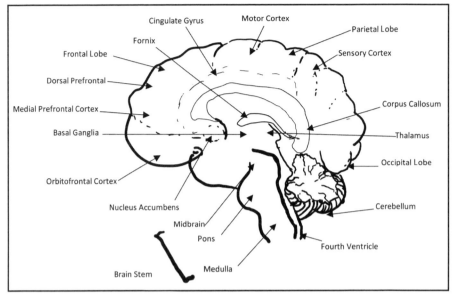

Figure 4-1. Midsagittal view of the brain with clear depiction of the dorsal, medial, and orbitofrontal areas; basal ganglia; and motor and sensory cortices.

goal-directed action. Thus, action possibilities are formed at multiple levels within these widespread systems and are enhanced or inhibited at different levels of the process to generate a specific response. Occupational adaptation heavily relies on the individual's ability to generate multiple action possibilities (adaptive response mechanisms; Schkade & Schultz, 1992) and the presence of healthy and accurate enhancing and inhibitory mechanisms for the final action selection. In the Occupational Adaptation (OA) model (Schkade & Schultz, 1992), this process is equivalent to specific adaptive response generation, evaluation, and integration processes.

Specific Brain Structures and Circuits

The *prefrontal cortex* is located in the anterior (front) of the brain and is part of the neocortex. Different areas in the prefrontal cortex differentially influence the action selection process. The prefrontal cortex is required for executive control of behavior (McGuire and Botvinick, 2010; Ridderinkhof, van Den Wildenberg, Segalowitz, & Carter, 2004) and for effective coping with stress (Amat et al., 2014; Sotres-Bayon & Quirk, 2010; Warden et al., 2012). Prefrontal dysfunction has been implicated in mood and anxiety disorders, which are typically associated with stressful life events (Etkin, Merhav, & Ordentlich, 2010; Mayberg et al., 1999; Milad & Quirk, 2012). Three main regions and related networks are distinguished for their differential contributions to action selection (Figure 4-1).

The *dorsolateral prefrontal* network involves the dorsolateral prefrontal regions (dorsal/upper region of the prefrontal lobe) that connect to sensory and motor association cortices, project to the basal ganglia, and receive input from substantia nigra. This network regulates the executive control of action based on semantic and perceptual information (Kandel et al., 2013). Injury to the dorsolateral prefrontal cortex results in cognitive deficits. For example, in a shopping trip where clear instructions are provided, a person with a focal dorsolateral lesion is unable to follow instructions, often breaks rules of social interaction, can be inefficient with task completion (i.e., following a sequence of prioritized steps), and usually fails to achieve intended outcomes. The individual perseverates on the use of inefficient strategies.

The *medial frontal cortex* and its network (below the dorsal prefrontal cortex) are essential to motivation (Kouneiher, Charron, & Koechlin, 2009). They monitor action selection based on the reward and emotional values of the action (Ridderinkhof, Ullsperger, Crone, & Nieuwenhuis, 2004; Jimura, Locke, & Braver, 2010). They have connections to the association cortices, thalamus, basal ganglia, and cingulate cortex (emotional brain circuit). These areas project to the amygdala (center for processing strong emotions such as fear) and the hypothalamus (regulation of homeostasis). Damage in the ventromedial system leads to impaired emotions and antisocial symptoms. Individuals with damage to this area do not present an emotional reaction when seeing pictures that usually provoke emotions (flat affect). These individuals are not reacting with changes in sympathetic activation before engaging in risky behavior or decisions (e.g., gambling). They are not good at making decisions under conditions of uncertainty in which reward and punishment are important. In any given interaction, they know social rules (intact dorsolateral prefrontal cortex) but fail to use them (Reber et al., 2017).

The *orbitofrontal network* is located at the base of the frontal region. It regulates impulses, compulsions, and internal/external drives. Specifically, it mediates homeostatic drives such as hunger, thirst, and mating through its connection to the hypothalamus, and it connects to the amygdala for regulation of fear and aggression (Kandel et al., 2013). This system projects and receives input from the dorsolateral prefrontal network. The communication regulates action decisions based on the control of impulse (Jonker, Jonker, Scheltens & Scherder, 2015). Damage to the orbital prefrontal cortex results in normal procedural cognitive skills (e.g., sequencing) but significant deficits in decision making. Deficits in this area relate to the inability to develop strategies that maximize the rewards within the context of tasks and inhibit impulses (Kandel et al., 2013; Grabenhorst & Rolls, 2011).

The *basal ganglia* is a constellation of subcortical structures. Most of the knowledge we have of this system is through studies of motor actions. The basal ganglia are known to influence the selection of motor action through their direct network connections to the motor cortex (Brown, Bullock, & Grossberg, 2004; Kalivas & Nakamura 1999; Leblois, Boraud, Meissner, Bergman, & Hansel, 2006; Mink, 1996). In addition, they are connected with the limbic system (emotional brain) and cortical regions such as the prefrontal cortex (Alexander & Crutcher, 1990; Middleton & Strick, 2000). The basal ganglia are associated with habitual action. Damaged connection of the ventral and dorsal basal ganglia regions is detected in obsessive-compulsive disorders. Damage in the dopaminergic network that regulates the function of the basal ganglia is central to Parkinson's disease.

The *amygdala* is involved in the regulation of emotion, particularly fear. Recently, it has been associated with processing of rewards as well (Kandel et al., 2013). Through its connection to the hippocampus system (memory processing system), it is involved in implicit regulation of action (unconscious recall and action selection based on the emotional value of prior experience).

The *anterior cingulate cortex* is part of the limbic system and significantly contributes to action. Through its connection to the prefrontal and parietal cortices, it regulates cognitive control of action selection. Through its connection to the amygdala, basal ganglia (nucleus accumbens), and hypothalamus, it is involved in detecting discrepancies between anticipated rewards and actual reward values of an action, contributing to error detection in action selection and motivational processes (Allman, Hakeem, Erwin, Nimchinsky, & Hof, 2001; Kandel et al., 2013).

Important Neurotransmitters and Hormones

The aforementioned areas communicate through chemical signals called *neurotransmitters*. Several neurotransmitters are involved in the planning and selection of action. Motivation and resilience influence actions through the neurochemical systems. In this chapter, we will focus on dopamine and stress-related neurochemical networks that lead to adaptive and maladaptive behaviors.

The *dopamine network* is the motivation network. It arises from two closely located but distinct regions: the substantia nigra and the ventral tegmental area in the midbrain. There are three pathways, the first two of which relate closely to the motivational and resilience components of action selection (Bromberg-Martin, Matsumoto, & Hikosaka, 2010):

- The *mesolimbic pathway*, in which neurons originate from the ventral tegmental area, regulates actions based on their reinforcement value. This system projects to the orbital and medial frontal cortex and basal ganglia (nucleus accumbens). It is thought to significantly contribute processes related to drug addiction.
- The *mesocortical pathway* also originates from the ventral tegmental area and supports the planning of action based on its emotional value (motivational properties of action) (Albrecht, Abeler, Weber, & Falk, 2014).
- The *nigrostriatal pathway* originates from the substantia nigra and connects to the basal ganglia. This system regulates movement initiation and execution.

The dopamine network regulates motivation for action in two distinct ways: the regulation of homeostasis and the modulation of the reward systems (Figure 4-2). *Regulation of homeostasis* includes satiation of basic survival needs such feeding, digestion, elimination, temperature, and maintenance of energy (Kandel et al., 2013). Modulation of rewards and consequences of action involves learning about the values of behaviors and actions. The dopaminergic reward system updates information for actions by generating a reward prediction error (RPE) from the difference between expected reward and experienced reward, thereby propagating learning through connections to the prefrontal cortex, amygdala, and ventral pallidum (basal ganglia). The mesolimbic and mesocortical dopamine networks support the process.

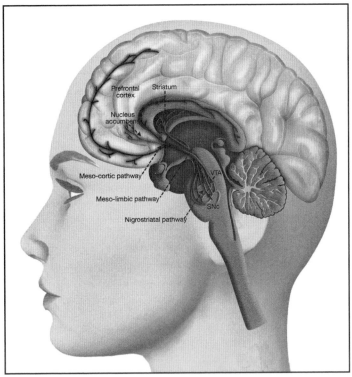

Figure 4-2. Dopaminergic system and reward processing. (Reprinted with permission from Arias-Carrión, O., Caraza-Santiago, X., Salgado-Licona, S., Salama, M., Machado S., Egidio Nardi, A., ... Murillo-Rodríguez, E. [2014]. Orquestic regulation of neurotransmitters on reward-seeking behavior. *International Archives of Medicine, 7,* 29. https://commons.wikimedia.org/wiki/File:Dopaminergic_system_and_reward_processing.jpg)

Current evidence suggests that dopamine neurons transmit in two modes. In the *tonic mode*, dopamine neurons maintain a steady baseline level, enabling the normal functions of neural circuits that they connect (Bromberg-Martin et al., 2010; Grace, Floresco, Goto, & Lodge, 2007; Schultz, 2007). In their *phasic mode*, dopamine neurons sharply increase or decrease their firing. This function helps to differentiate between actions that are highly motivating (increased reward value) vs not motivating (decreased reward value).

Additional projections of the dopamine network to the nucleus accumbens (basal ganglia) relate to activation under not just pleasure-related rewards, but also effort-related estimates (Phillips, Walton, & Jhou, 2007; Rushworth, Walton, Kennerley, & Bannerman, 2004; Salamone, Correa, Mingote, & Weber, 2003). This area of research examines the selection of action based on the cost-benefit ratio (effort ratio). It encompasses cognitive processes as well as somatic and autonomic system responses. Simpson and Balsam (2016) discuss the idea that the motivational drive is influenced by the individual's processing of both the benefits and the costs related to any action or behavior.

The benefits related to behavioral action might include fulfilling psychological or physiological needs, obtaining reinforcement secondary to those needs, or escaping from or avoiding harm or punishment. The costs associated with behavioral action include physical or mental effort, time, potential discomfort or danger, and loss of potential opportunities. In any action, the value of every cost and every benefit is calculated, encoded, and processed relative to the individual's physiological state as well as contextual information. Then, when the goal is obtained, the result and the cost-benefit value are stored for future retrieval when obtaining that goal again becomes relevant (Simpson & Balsam, 2016).

Furthermore, motivation to carry out a specific action seems to be affected by whether the task at hand requires cognitive or physical effort. Schmidt, Lebreton, Cléry-Melin, Daunizeau, and Pessiglione (2012) investigated the neural mechanisms for the motivation of cognitive vs physical efforts for tasks. Cognitive effort is processed through a connection from the ventral prefrontal cortex to the ventral striatum (basal ganglia). Motivation for physical effort is mainly processed through the limbic system and basal ganglia (mostly the ventral striatum and pallidum), with primary connections to the motor cortex. Schmidt et al. (2012) investigated whether cognitive and physical efforts are controlled or driven by a common, generic motivational process or whether cognitive and physical efforts are driven by distinct, dedicated systems. Results of their research indicate that motivation for rewarded behavior or action is encoded in the ventral striatum (basal ganglia). The ventral striatum can then drive either the motor or cognitive part of the dorsal striatum, depending on the task. A connection between the ventral striatum and the dorsal striatum is common for the motivation of cognitive and physical effort in a task or goal-directed behavior.

Stress Neurochemical Networks and the Neurobiology of Resilience

Resilience refers to physiological and behavioral adaptation to stressors. From a physiological perspective, resilience refers to mechanisms that support survival and well-being. Neural systems have a propensity for homeostasis (Kandel et al., 2013). *Homeostasis* is the maintenance of biophysiological conditions that must be preserved to ensure survival and well-being. The body makes constant modifications to respond to and counteract stressors that could disturb homeostasis. The term *allostasis* describes the dynamic regulation and maintenance of homeostasis (Ramsay & Woods, 2014; Sterling & Eyer, 1988) and refers to the process by which, in order to survive and function, organisms need to be able to change physiologically to adjust to the new and changing environments. For example, to cope with an unexpected stressor, an individual might maintain an elevated level of blood pressure. The process creates an *allostatic load*, which is the physiological result or cost of adaptation to stressors (McEwen, 2008). The capacity of the allostatic load is a measure of the brain's ability to resume its pre-allostatic state and is inversely proportional to the degree of resilience. In our previous example, prolonged periods of elevated level of blood pressure can cause damage that can be irreversible. In this context, resilience is the ability of the central nervous system and the body to minimize allostatic load and successfully adapt to stressors. Gavidia-Payne, Denny, Davis,

Francis, and Jackson (2015) hypothesized that resilience is a form of biophysiological adaptation. Long-term stress and impairments pose significant demands on the neural systems to adapt. Lack of adaptation can lead to myriad health issues, including increased vulnerability to hypertension, immunosuppression, osteoporosis, insulin resistance, truncal obesity, cardiovascular disease, anxiety, depressive disorders, and post-traumatic stress disorder (PTSD) (Carroll et al., 2007; Whitworth & Aichhorn, 2005; Glaser & Kiecolt-Glaser, 2005). Further research on the neurobiology of resilience has focused on the following neurochemical mechanisms: serotonin receptors, neuropeptide Y, and the hypothalamic-pituitary-adrenal (HPA) axis (Kandel et al., 2013; Russo, Murrough, Han, Charney, & Nestler, 2012).

Serotonin Receptors (5-HT)

During moments or times of stress, cortisol (a steroid-based hormone) is released from the adrenal cortex within the adrenal gland. The response to cortisol is arousal, attention, and memory formation, as well as increased blood glucose and blood pressure and suppressed immune processes. In contrast, serotonin, or 5-hydroxytryptamine (5-HT), a monoamine neurotransmitter, is thought to be a contributor to feelings of well-being and happiness. Serotonergic receptive neurons are found throughout the central nervous system and modulate the release of many neurotransmitters, including glutamate, gamma-aminobutyric acid (GABA), dopamine, epinephrine/norepinephrine, and acetylcholine. The serotonin receptors impact various biological and neurological processes, including modulating appetite, mood, and thermoregulation; decreasing aggression, anxiety, and nausea; and increasing cognition, learning, memory, and sleep. Maintaining lower levels of cortisol and other stress-induced neurochemicals and maintaining higher levels of serotonin receptor activity contributes to resilience and adaptive response to stress.

Neuropeptide Y

Neuropeptide Y is a peptide neurotransmitter that appears to modulate stress responses in animals. Studies in humans support the possibility that neuropeptide Y may represent a protective factor in the face of stress. Specifically, neuropeptide Y is thought to limit the stress response by reducing sympathetic nervous system activation and protecting the brain from the harmful effects of chronically elevated cortisol levels. Morgan, Rasmusson, Wang, Hoyt, Hauger, and Hazlett (2002) found that higher blood neuropeptide Y levels predicted better performance during stressful military survival training and specifically that higher levels of neuropeptide Y were found in Special Forces soldiers compared with non–Special Forces military counterparts. The researchers reported that higher levels of neuropeptide Y in response to acute stress resulted in less psychological distress and fewer stress symptoms (Morgan et al., 2002). This study suggests a protective role for neuropeptide Y under conditions of high stress, which is consistent with tentative human genetic studies that weakly implicate variations in the neuropeptide Y gene in emotional behavior and stress responses (Mickey et al., 2011; Morgan et al., 2000; Zhou et al., 2008).

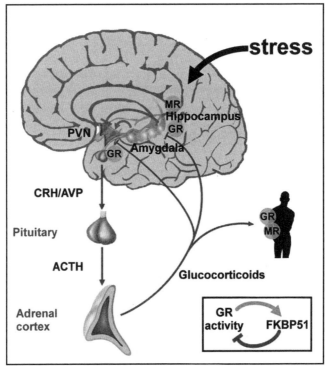

Figure 4-3. The HPA axis mediates stress responses. The periventricular nucleus (PVN) at the hypothalamus can magnify the intensity of the stressor via feedback from the hippocampus and amygdala. Mineralocorticoid (MR) receptors start the stress response while glucocorticoid receptors (GR) can terminate the stress response. Hypothalamic neuropeptides corticotrophin-releasing hormone (CRH) and arginine vasopressin (AVP) promote the synthesis and secretion of adrenocorticotrophin (ACTH). ACTH in turn stimulates the release of glucocorticoids from the adrenal glands. These hormones travel throughout the body and the brain and connect to steroid receptors in the cells. The GR also activate a protein (FKBP51) that reduces GR activity within the cells. (Reprinted with permission from Raabe, F. J., & Spengler, D. [2013]. Epigenetic risk factors in PTSD and depression. *Frontiers in Psychiatry, 4*, 80. https://commons. wikimedia.org/wiki/File:Hypothalamic-pituitary-adrenal_axis.jpg)

The Hypothalamus-Pituitary-Adrenal Axis

A primary mediator of the influence of stress on the central nervous system and behavior is activation of the HPA axis, which results in widespread hormonal, neurochemical, and physiological alterations in the brain and body (Herman & Cullinan, 1997; Ozbay, Fitterling, Charney, & Southwick, 2008). The HPA axis comprises the hypothalamus, pituitary, and adrenal glands, which are the primary hormonal processors of the body (Figure 4-3). As a result of stress, the HPA axis is activated, resulting in widespread hormonal, neurochemical, and physiological brain adjustments (Herman & Cullinan,

1997), specifically the release of glucocorticoids from the adrenal cortex. Glucocorticoids interact with steroid receptors throughout the brain and function primarily to regulate cellular function beyond the time scale of acute stress effects. Glucocorticoid receptors and other receptors are expressed at high levels in the hippocampus, amygdala, medial prefrontal cortex, and other limbic and midbrain structures. In these structures of the central nervous system, the glucocorticoids modulate the neural circuitry that underlies behavioral responses to stress.

As mentioned, the hippocampus is one of the primary brain structures that exerts strong regulatory control over the HPA axis. In studies with humans and with rats, stimulation of the hippocampus decreases glucocorticoid secretion. Yet a lesion of the hippocampus elevates the basal glucocorticoid level, especially during the stress recovery phase (Jankord & Herman, 2008). In humans, disorders of glutamatergic neurotransmission, structural maladaptive and functional changes in the circuitry of the hippocampus, and decreased hippocampal volume have been associated with stress-related conditions such as major depressive disorder (Sanacora, Treccani, & Popoli, 2012).

Complex neural processes underlie adaptation. Neural networks regulate physiological and functional adaptation in a dynamic pattern to accommodate flexible interaction between the person and the environmental and task demands. Goal-directed actions are regulated by intent and motivational systems that shift the physiological state of the entire brain and body. Resilience is the process that supports homeostatic balance and regulates adaptation to preserve overall health and wellness. Tasks, occupations, and environments generate physiological and behavioral responses and trigger adaptation. However, internal neurobiological changes may also require adaptation. For example, growth and development pose significant challenges for adaptation. Babies have to constantly adapt to a growing body and significantly modify their actions to accomplish their goals. Occupational adaptation is a critical neurobiological process of change to support the dynamic fit between a person's biological and psychological state and his or her meaningful activities and occupations.

NEUROBIOLOGICAL CHANGES AND THE PROCESS OF OCCUPATIONAL ADAPTATION

Occupational adaptation involves complex neural processes in response to changes and challenges within an individual's life. In this section, we will review developmental changes in conjunction with early experiences that shape neural processes related to occupational adaptation, and we will examine changes in health as a result of lifestyle choices, trauma, or prolonged exposure to stress and their impact on neural networks and their capacity for adaptation. Finally, we will review the processes of neuroplastic conditions that facilitate occupational adaptation and the ability to cope with adversity or trauma, thus influencing the recovery process.

Adaptive Changes Due to Growth and Development

As mentioned in Chapter 3, development of the adaptive neural systems is gradual; it starts in infancy and continues into young adulthood until approximately 25 years old (Gogtay et al., 2004). The gradual nature of this development process emphasizes the interactive nature of these adaptive neural systems with personal experiences. One could argue that adaptive neural systems are geared toward individual preferences in occupational engagement within the context of diverse environments. It also signifies the vulnerability of the adaptive neural systems to stressors and their impact on development. Goal-directed action and control of action, as regulated by the development of the prefrontal cortex, has monopolized the literature. Basic processes of executive functioning develop rapidly in the early childhood years (4 to 6 years old, primarily), with another period of increased plasticity during the transition to adolescence (Andrews-Hanna, 2012; Cantlon et al., 2011). These changes manifest themselves in adaptive behaviors during task demands that require flexible control of attention. For example, at 4 years old, attention can switch between two sets of rules (e.g., "hold the ball with two hands and throw it at the target" or "sit down during circle time and listen to a story") if instructed. Early executive control is externally driven; that is, children need to be told what the rules are, and they tend to perseverate on self-initiated goals. The gradual maturation for the prefrontal cortex originates in the orbitofrontal area and progresses toward the dorsal and rostral areas of cortex (Zelazo & Carlson, 2012). The control of impulses and regulation of homeostasis precede the control of emotional selection of action, which precede the executive control of action (Bunge & Wright, 2007; Johnson, Munro, & Bunge, 2014). Age-related changes continue to be observed between 8 and 17 years old (Bunge & Zelazo, 2006). For example, when comparing 5- to 7-year-olds to 9- to 11-year-olds in an action inhibition task (e.g., release the home key and press the target key), older children were able to stop a motor plan earlier in the execution phase than younger children (Johnstone et al., 2007).

What Are the Developmental, Genetic, and Environmental Factors That Contribute to Plasticity?

In this section, we present the process in typically developing children. One plausible explanation is the gradual myelination process (Gogtay et al., 2004). The child and adolescent brain undergoes substantial myelination and white matter growth. Cortical reorganization and cortical thinning (i.e., long-range connections such as the dopamine networks are formed across distant brain regions and overrule local networks) are also critical. However, we will argue that occupational engagement and adaptation to task and activity demands with increased complexity guide this process of adaptive development. The newborn baby is caught in consistent and habitual patterns of interaction with the environment with little variability in action possibilities. The first level of control toward more flexible behavioral responses involves the ability to overcome habitual action and increase the response to changing environmental demands. Enriched motivating environments are conducive to more exploration (information gathering) and more interaction with tasks. The changing environmental demands and rapidly changing bodies create an ideal context for the process of occupational adaptation and the development of neural structures to support it (Als et al., 2004; Johnson, 2001).

The second level of control entails the need to set goals and motivation to achieve these goals that leads to proactive control of action rather than reactive control (Bunge & Wright, 2007). As the environment becomes more than the toddler's house and walking radically expands access to novel and ambiguous tasks, proactive control of action is a result and a necessity in this process.

Finally, intentional behavior and goal-directed actions within more complex environments introduce variability that leads to learning of sophisticated response parameters and attempts to generalize the successful behavior and outcome into novel situations. The emergence of the motivation to initiate action that is more self-directed is evident. The neural connections that we see in mature systems begin to form under this drive and create the conditions for proactive control of action selection and action execution.

Children and adults differ in the efficiency of action while solving possible problems. For example, children appear to update rules related to the action prediction and selection slower than adults (Ezekiel, Bosma, & Morton, 2013). However, there is evidence of both systems being able to solve possible problems using different neural structures. In a recent study, Ezekiel et al. (2013) tested children in middle childhood and adults using a card sort/switch cognitive control task. Adults used the dorsolateral prefrontal cortex, medial prefrontal cortex, anterior cingulate cortex, inferior parietal cortex, and ventral tegmental area. In children, they observed activation of the anterior frontal gyrus, rostral prefrontal cortex, anterior insula (emotional circuit, mostly on the right side), and left posterior temporal cortex (associated with language). The study indicates that adults use more executive function decision-making motivation networks to solve these problems (faster approach), whereas children use more social-emotional and language-based networks to solve the same problems (slower process).

The role of genetic factors in the developmental process of adaptive action is less understood. Studies have linked cognitive control and dopamine networks and suggest that the interaction between genes and environment influences the rate of development in functions that are relevant such as self-regulation. Genetic maps support complex heritability of white matter integrity, cortical thickness, and intelligence quotient (IQ). Lenroot et al. (2009) investigated age-related differences in the heritability of cortical thickness using magnetic resonance imaging (MRI) with a large pediatric sample of twins, twin siblings, and singletons (n = 600; mean age, 11.1 years). The primary sensory and motor cortex show greater genetic effects earlier in childhood. Later-developing regions within the dorsal prefrontal cortex (e.g., tool use, executive function) and temporal lobes (e.g., language) conversely show increasingly prominent genetic effects with maturation. These higher cognitive functions appear more heritable in adolescents than in children (Plomin, Fulker, Corley, & DeFries, 1997).

Cognitive and emotional systems continue to adapt in adulthood. Education, social interaction, and active engagement in meaningful occupations are significant predictors of health and well-being and the support of productive aging (Stern, 2009). The theoretical model of cognitive reserve suggests that individual differences in the cognitive processes that relate to task performance allow some adults to cope better than others with brain damage, trauma, or mental decline due to the aging process. For example, in an epidemiological study, increased literacy (as part of the active engagement in the educational process) was associated with slower decline in memory, executive function, and language skills in community-dwelling older adults (Manly, Touradji, Tang, & Stern, 2003).

Body changes and environmental demands guide the development and refinement of neural processes of adaptation (cognitive and emotional networks). Although there are clearly periods that have more possibilities for growth and development, positive engagement in meaningful tasks throughout life promotes flexibility and endurance in these systems.

IMPACT OF STRESS IN THE OCCUPATIONAL ADAPTATION PROCESS

Stressors Can Impose a Maladaptive Neural Process

Stressors can be psychological and biological and can have a different impact on the adaptation process depending on the developmental or homeostatic state of the individual. Biological factors can impact the process of adaptation and promote health or disease. Genetic predisposition to specific protein production can control chronic stress responses and can lead to either exaggerated or very mild responses to stress. In addition, biological differences in gene interaction with specific environmental conditions (epigenetic process) can lead to adaptive or maladaptive responses to stressors. Then, experiences from the interactions with the world can shape the neural and neurochemical structure of the brain, especially early in life. Specifically, positive experiences increase the connectivity of adaptive neural networks that promote positive emotions and actions and increase the productive presence of dopamine for active engagement in goal-directed action. Finally, biological stressors such as inflammation (as an autoimmune response or lifestyle) can impact the process of adaptation. Chronic inflammation can lead to serious disease (e.g., arthritis, cancer, diabetes). Taking action to decrease biological stressors increases the body's ability to adapt to changing demands of occupations and promotes health.

Vulnerable Developmental Periods

Some developmental periods, such as the prenatal period, early childhood, and adolescence, are considered more vulnerable than middle childhood or adulthood (Heim & Binder, 2012). We present two examples of stressors (one psychological and one biological) and their impact in the adaptive process. The first example refers to prolonged exposure to psychological stress. Epidemiological studies suggest that prenatal exposure to stress (such as mother's depression) or to excess glucocorticoids increases the risk for low birth weight or small size at birth and is associated with neurophysiological changes affecting the infant's ability to regulate stress (high cortisol levels and HPA axis activation), with consequences for mental health problems in adulthood (Seckl & Holmes, 2007). Early childhood exposure to stressors has been associated with increased prevalence of depression and mood and anxiety disorders in adolescence and adulthood (Heim & Binder, 2012; Sirin & Rogers-Sirin, 2015). For example, McCauley et al. (1997) studied 1900 women and found that childhood sexual or physical abuse was associated with increases in symptoms of depression and anxiety, addiction, psychiatric admissions, and suicide attempts.

Adolescence is another sensitive period because the hormonal changes lead to already elevated levels of stress. An array of mental health problems have their onset during this period, including depression and anxiety disorders. Changes in the neural integrity of the frontal cortex and reduced size in the anterior cingulate cortex are evident in adolescents with a history of abuse (Heim & Binder, 2012). Exposure to prolonged stressful conditions during the critical periods can have a lifelong negative impact to the individual's occupational adaptation process.

The second example relates to a biological stressor exposure during vulnerable developmental periods. Although the etiology of schizophrenia remains unknown, an increasing body of evidence suggests that prenatal and perinatal exposure to infections (e.g., influenza, rubella) as well as immune response to infections contribute to an increased risk of developing schizophrenia later in life (Heim & Binder, 2012). Neuroimaging studies confirm that during the same developmental periods, there is a widespread gray matter loss across cortical regions that is more pronounced in the prefrontal cortical area (Heim & Binder, 2012). The actual manifestation of the disease occurs in the adolescent years as a consequence of the overall synaptic pruning process that occurs during that time (Sørensen, Mortensen, Reinisch, & Mednick, 2009).

Vulnerable Homeostatic State: Examples of Stressors Affecting Homeostatic States of Adults

The homeostatic state of the individual at the time of exposure to stress can alter the severity of the consequences and impact the recovery process. For example, a robust number of studies report prolonged elevated glucocorticoid levels in individuals with depression, stress, and anxiety disorders. The altered homeostatic state of these individuals can then influence their preferences and their ability to cope with further stress and life experiences (Armstrong & Olatunji, 2012). Hereditary characteristics can create vulnerable homeostatic conditions to stressors and trauma in adulthood. For example, a twin study of Vietnam veterans suggested that the decreased hippocampal volume (hereditary factor) was evident in those exposed to trauma compared to those who had no exposure, thus considering the hippocampal volume a risk factor for PTSD. Decreased hippocampal volume increased the vulnerability to stress and trauma (Gilbertson et al., 2002). Early prolonged exposure to stressors can alter the adaptability of the person to adverse conditions later in life.

Creating Conditions for Recovery

The process of occupational adaptation signifies the ability to overcome challenges and can partially explain why some individuals fare better than others when faced with adverse life events or biological stressors. For example, some children who faced significant adversity early in life have productive lives. Increasing evidence suggests that individual (health and genetic factors) and environmental factors dynamically influence a person's ability for occupational adaptation.

Behavioral factors that interface with neural networks can support the adaptive process with significant positive consequences for health and well-being in response to trauma and adversity. Here we present principles and strategies that support the process of occupational engagement and promote neural and behavior adaptation toward health and wellness (Shonkoff et al., 2015). Behavioral intervention studies that have systematically examined the effects of specific principles related to resilience and a positive adaptive process are scarce. Even fewer studies have traced the effects of behavioral interventions and their neural network impact. Existing evidence presented here constitutes examples of the evidence needed to support strategies of successful adaptation and recovery in response to adversity and trauma (Shonkoff et al., 2015):

- Increasing self-awareness and control of the health process, so that the individual maintains or regains control of the adaptive behaviors and habits. Neurobiological systems of motivation and executive function support this process and restore or create neural networks that can generate possibilities for action, and thus flexibility (Shonkoff et al., 2015). For occupational therapy, age-appropriate activities embedded in meaningful occupations significantly improve the potential for recovery and restoration. Occupational therapy programs that actively build skills based on interest, encourage planning and organization, address impulse control, and promote cognitive flexibility have a significant impact on promoting the adaptive process. The following is an example of a behavioral intervention called Training in Awareness, Resilience, and Action (TARA), which was developed to target specific mechanisms in adolescent depression (Henje Blom et al., 2017). TARA comprises training of autonomic (to address amygdala hyperactivation) and emotional self-regulation (notice negative references about self and rephrase), interoceptive awareness (increase awareness, especially those related to autonomic reactions), relational skills, and value-based committed action. A preliminary single-arm clinical trial was conducted with 26 adolescents (14 to 18 years old) diagnosed with depression participating in a 12-week group program. Significant changes in overall symptomatology of depression and anxiety were reported immediately after the intervention and at 3-month follow-up (Henje Blom et al., 2017).
- Building a sense of purpose and mastery over activities and life circumstances. The process of adaptation is strengthened by the accumulation of successful and meaningful experiences. Rewarding, supportive environments can facilitate the process. In a study of college students who reported heavy drinking within the past 6 months, increased engagement and participation in meaningful, rewarding activities was associated with lower likelihood of alcohol consumption (Turner & Johnson, 2003). In another study of individuals with depression and a history of alcohol abuse, activity enjoyment and not frequency was associated with the decrease in alcohol consumption. Supportive systems and environments that consistently promote health habits and meaningful exchanges can counterbalance the influence of the disease through a bottom-up process of positive experience and mastery (Turner & Johnson, 2003).

- Stable, caring, supportive relationships trigger the activation of positive emotional states and create conditions for selection and execution of adaptive actions. Evidence from studies on military veterans supports the link between social support systems and resilience resulting in mental health. For example, in a study that collected cross-sectional data from veterans who presented resilience in the face of traumatic experiences, they had more social supports (e.g., they were married or living with a partner) and scored higher in social connectedness measures and community engagement than those with higher signs of distress (Pietrzak & Cook, 2013).

- Contextual supports through cultural and spiritual traditions increase the possibility of effective coping with adversity and trauma. Emotional and cognitive supports of cultural systems are embedded in the decision-making process and strengthen the choice of adaptive actions that promote health vs disease (Masten, 2014).

CASE STUDY: ADAM Adam is 25 years old who experienced a blast injury while serving in Afghanistan with the U.S. Army. The injury resulted in a bilateral upper extremity amputation. Following rehabilitation, he lost interest in most of the activities he previously enjoyed and experienced night terrors. His wife, Ashley, reported that he spent most days watching television or sleeping. He returned to rehabilitation for advanced prosthetic fitting and training. At that time, he was diagnosed with PTSD, anxiety, and depression. Adam worked with his occupational therapist, Steve, to identify his interests and hobbies. Initially, he was not able to identify many interests other than typical activities of daily living (e.g., brushing his teeth, washing his own hair, making his own coffee). He expressed that it was demoralizing to ask Ashley for help for everything.

Slowly, Adam became more proficient with the use of his prostheses. Adam and Steve worked together daily to identify activities that were meaningful to him. One day, he mentioned that as a boy he used to ride horses competitively. Steve told him about an equine program for veterans that included hippotherapy, grooming, sports riding, and vaulting. Several months after discharge, Adam contacted Steve. He told him that he was grooming horses daily with the equine program. He was beginning to learn competitive barrel racing. He also excitedly told Steve that he and Ashley were now engaged. Although Adam admitted that he still struggled with PTSD and had some bad days, he was able to cope overall and looked forward to his future.

Adam's case provides an example of occupation-based programming to support occupational adaptation. Creating conditions for recovery from adversity and health challenges is difficult but necessary to support occupational adaptation. Experiences that increase awareness of health and give the person control of his or her actions in conjunction with a sense of mastery and purpose can impact the process of adaptation. Environments that provide support to personal growth are important for sustainable results. The process of occupational adaptation has neurobiological underpinnings. Conditions that support adaptation and recovery are necessary for sustainable results.

ADVANCING THE KNOWLEDGE ON OCCUPATIONAL ADAPTATION

The neurobiological processes underlying intention and goal-directed action provide a primary adaptive capacity via flexible alternative possibilities for occupational engagement. Motivation and resilience are key processes that can create conditions of positive adaptation to reverse the consequence of trauma or adversity. This chapter has provided insights regarding processes of positive and negative adaptation, with strong supports that the nature of experiences and active engagement of the individual are critical for the process of adaptation. Occupational adaptation reflects the behavioral manifestation of these process and closely relates to neural network functions. By understanding these processes and the factors that affect adaptation, occupational therapists can incorporate science-driven strategy to improve interventions in the context of occupational adaptations. Additionally, the occupational therapy practitioner can create an environment in which adaptive behaviors become learned skills. In return, the client takes an active part in the therapy process, contributing to the success of his or her own treatment. The responsibility of taking charge of one's health and well-being is reinforced through a cooperative process by allowing the client to witness his or her own motivation, intention, goal-directed behaviors, and resilience. Through this partnership, both the occupational therapy practitioner and the client validate the creative engagement that has occurred and the expectation that future adaptations can take place.

SUMMARY AND IMPLICATIONS

- Adaptation is a complex neurobiological process that involves several networks. Decision making and motivational networks are major underlying mechanisms to understand the process of adaptation.
- Evidence suggests that development and exposure to stressors (biological and/or behavioral) significantly affect the ability and direction of the adaptive process.
- Neurobiological and behavioral studies support that promoting awareness, control, and a sense of mastery in a person and creating supportive environments can trigger the adaptive process and support positive changes in the brain that translate to function.
- The link between how occupational engagement and adaptation can alter neurobiological processes has gain increased interest in the scientific and clinical research. More studies are needed in this area.

REFERENCES

Albrecht, K., Abeler, J., Weber, B., & Falk, A. (2014). The brain correlates of the effects of monetary and verbal rewards on intrinsic motivation. *Frontiers in Neuroscience, 8*, 303.

Alexander, G. E., & Crutcher, M. D. (1990). Functional architecture of basal ganglia circuits: Neural substrates of parallel processing. *Trends in Neurosciences, 13*, 266-271.

Allman, J. M., Hakeem, A., Erwin, J. M., Nimchinsky, E., & Hof, P. (2001). The anterior cingulate cortex. The evolution of an interface between emotion and cognition. *Annals of the New York Academy of Sciences, 935*(1), 107-117.

Als, H., Duffy, F. H., McAnulty, G. B., Rivkin, M. J., Vajapeyam, S., Mulkern, R. V., … Eichenwald, E. C. (2004). Early experience alters brain function and structure. *Pediatrics, 113*(4), 846-857.

Amat, J., Christianson, J. P., Aleksejev, R. M., Kim, J., Richeson, K. R., Watkins, L. R., & Maier, S. F. (2014). Control over a stressor involves the posterior dorsal striatum and the act/outcome circuit. *European Journal of Neuroscience, 40*(2), 2352-2358.

Andrews-Hanna, J. R. (2012). The brain's default network and its adaptive role in internal mentation. *The Neuroscientist, 18*(3), 251-270. doi:10.1177/1073858411403316

Armstrong, T., & Olatunji, B. O. (2012). Eye tracking of attention in the affective disorders: A meta-analytic review and synthesis. *Clinical Psychology Review, 32*(8), 704-723.

Balleine, B. W., and O'Doherty, J. P. (2010). Human and rodent homologies in action control: Cortico-striatal determinants of goal-directed and habitual action. *Neuropsychopharmacology, 35*(1), 48-69.

Belujon, P., & Grace, A. A. (2015). Regulation of dopamine system responsivity and its adaptive and pathological response to stress. *Biological Sciences, 282*(1805).

Bromberg-Martin, E. S., Matsumoto, M., & Hikosaka, O. (2010). Dopamine in motivational control: Rewarding, aversive, and alerting. *Neuron, 68*(5), 815-834.

Brown, J. W., Bullock, D., & Grossberg, S. (2004). How laminar frontal cortex and basal ganglia circuits interact to control planned and reactive saccades. *Neural Networks, 17*(4), 471-510.

Bunge, S. A., & Wright, S. B. (2007). Neurodevelopmental changes in working memory and cognitive control. *Current Opinion in Neurobiology, 17*(2), 243-250.

Bunge, S. A., & Zelazo, P. D. (2006). A brain-based account of the development of rule use in childhood. *Current Directions in Psychological Science, 15*(3), 118-121.

Cantlon, J. F., Davis, S. W., Libertus, M. E., Kahane, J., Brannon, E. M., & Pelphrey, K. A. (2011). Interparietal white matter development predicts numerical performance in young children. *Learning and Individual Differences, 21*(6), 672-680. doi:10.1016/j.lindif.2011.09.003

Cao, J. L., Covington, H. E., Friedman, A. K., Wilkinson, M. B., Walsh, J. J., Cooper, D. C., … Han, M. H. (2010). Mesolimbic dopamine neurons in the brain reward circuit mediate susceptibility to social defeat and antidepressant action. *Journal of Neuroscience, 30*(49), 16453-16458.

Carroll, B. J., Cassidy, F., Naftolowitz, D., Tatham, N. E., Wilson, W. H., Iranmanesh, A., … Veldhuis, J. D. (2007). Pathophysiology of hypercortisolism in depression. *Acta Psychiatrica Scandinavica, 115*(Suppl.433), 90-103.

Cisek, P. (2007). Cortical mechanisms of action selection: The affordance competition hypothesis. *Philosophical Transactions of the Royal Society B: Biological Sciences, 362*(1485), 1585-1599.

Cisek, P., & Kalaska, J. F. (2010). Neural mechanisms for interacting with a world full of action choices. *Annual Review of Neuroscience, 33*, 269-298.

Etkin, R. H., Merhav, N., & Ordentlich, E. (2010). Error exponents of optimum decoding for the interference channel. *IEEE Transactions on Information Theory, 56*(1), 40-56.

Ezekiel, F., Bosma, R., & Morton, J. B. (2013). Dimensional change card sort performance associated with age-related differences in functional connectivity of lateral prefrontal cortex. *Developmental Cognitive Neuroscience, 5*, 40-50.

Fine, S. B. (1991). Resilience and human adaptability: Who rises above adversity? *American Journal of Occupational Therapy, 45*(6), 493-503.

Frankl, V. E. (1959). *From death-camp to existentialism: A psychiatrist's path to a new therapy.* Boston, MA: Beacon Press.

Gavidia-Payne, S., Denny, B., Davis, K., Francis, A., & Jackson, M. (2015). Parental resilience: A neglected construct in resilience research. *Clinical Psychologist, 19*(3), 111-121. doi:10.1111/cp.12053

Gilbertson, M. W., Shenton, M. E., Ciszewski, A., Kasai, K., Lasko, N. B., Orr, S. P., & Pitman, R. K. (2002). Smaller hippocampal volume predicts pathologic vulnerability to psychological trauma. *Nature Neuroscience, 5*(11), 1242-1247.

Glaser, R., & Kiecolt-Glaser, J. K. (2005). Stress-induced immune dysfunction: Implications for health. *Nature Reviews Immunology, 5*(3), 243-251.

Gogtay, N., Giedd, J. N., Lusk, L., Hayashi, K. M., Greenstein, D., Vaituzis, A. C., ... Thompson, P. M. (2004). Dynamic mapping of human cortical development during childhood through early adulthood. *Proceedings of the National Academy of Sciences of the United States of America, 101*(21), 8174-8179.

Grabenhorst, F., & Rolls, E. T. (2011). Value, pleasure and choice in the ventral prefrontal cortex. *Trends in Cognitive Sciences, 15*(2), 56-67.

Grace, A. A., Floresco, S. B., Goto, Y., & Lodge, D. J. (2007). Regulation of firing of dopaminergic neurons and control of goal-directed behaviors. *Trends in Neurosciences, 30*(5), 220-227.

Grajo, L. C. (2017). Occupational adaptation. In J. Hinojosa, P. Kramer, & C. Royeen (Eds.), *Perspectives on human occupations: Theories underlying practice* (pp. 287-312). Philadelphia, PA: F. A. Davis.

Hare, T. A., Camerer, C. F., & Rangel, A. (2009). Self-control in decision-making involves modulation of the vmPFC valuation system. *Science, 324*(5927), 646-648.

Heim, C., & Binder, E. B. (2012). Current research trends in early life stress and depression: Review of human studies on sensitive periods, gene-environment interactions, and epigenetics. *Experimental Neurology, 233*(1), 102-111.

Henje Blom, E., Tymofiyeva, O., Chesney, M. A., Ho, T. C., Moran, P., Connolly, C. G., ... Yang, T. T. (2017). Feasibility and preliminary efficacy of a novel rDoc-based treatment program for adolescent depression: "Training for Awareness Resilience and Action" (TARA)—A pilot study. *Frontiers in Psychiatry, 7,* 208.

Herman J. P., & Cullinan W. E. (1997). Neurocircuitry of stress: Central control of the hypothalamo-pituitary-adrenocortical axis. *Trends in Neurosciences, 20,* 78-84.

Jankord, R., & Herman, J. P. (2008). Limbic regulation of hypothalamo-pituitary-adrenocortical function during acute and chronic stress. *Annals of the New York Academy of Sciences, 1148*(1), 64-73.

Jimura, K., Locke, H., & Braver, T. (2010). Prefrontal cortex mediation of cognitive enhancement in rewarding motivational contexts. *Proceedings of the National Academy of Sciences of the United States of America, 107,* 8871-8876.

Johnson, E. L., Munro, S. E., & Bunge, S. A. (2014). Development of neural networks supporting goal-directed behavior. In P. D. Zelazo & M. D. Sera (Eds.), *Minnesota Symposia on Child Psychology: Developing cognitive control processes: Mechanisms, implications, and interventions* (Vol. 37, pp. 21-54). Hoboken, NJ: John Wiley & Sons.

Johnson, M. H. (2001). Functional brain development in humans. *Nature Reviews Neuroscience, 2*(7), 475-483.

Johnstone, S. J., Dimoska, A., Smith, J. L., Barry, R. J., Pleffer, C. B., Chiswick, D., & Clarke, A. R. (2007). The development of stop-signal and Go/Nogo response inhibition in children aged 7-12 years: Performance and event-related potential indices. *International Journal of Psychophysiology, 63*(1), 25-38.

Jonker, F. A., Jonker, C., Scheltens, P., & Scherder, E. J. (2015). The role of the orbitofrontal cortex in cognition and behavior. *Reviews in the Neurosciences, 26*(1), 1-11. doi:10.1515/revneuro-2014-0043

Kahnt, T., Park, S. Q., Cohen, M. X., Beck, A., Heinz, A., & Wrase, J. (2009). Dorsal striatal-midbrain connectivity in humans predicts how reinforcements are used to guide decisions. *Journal of Cognitive Neuroscience, 21*(7), 1332-1345. doi:10.1162/jocn.2009.21092

Kalivas, P. W., & Nakamura, M. (1999). Neural systems for behavioral activation and reward. *Current Opinion in Neurobiology, 9*(2), 223-227.

Kandel, E. R., Schwartz, J. H., Jessell, T. M., Siegelbaum, S. A., & Hudspeth, A. J. (Eds.). (2013). *Principles of neural science* (5th ed.). New York, NY: McGraw-Hill.

Kouneiher, F., Charron, S., & Koechlin, E. (2009). Motivation and cognitive control in the human prefrontal cortex. *Nature Neuroscience, 12*(7), 939-945.

Leblois, A., Boraud, T., Meissner, W., Bergman, H., & Hansel, D. (2006). Competition between feedback loops underlies normal and pathological dynamics in the basal ganglia. *Journal of Neuroscience, 26*(13), 3567-3583.

Lenroot, R. K., Schmitt, J. E., Ordaz, S. J., Wallace, G. L., Neale, M. C., Lerch, J. P., … Giedd, J. N. (2009). Differences in genetic and environmental influences on the human cerebral cortex associated with development during childhood and adolescence. *Human Brain Mapping, 30*(1), 163-174.

Leung, B. K., & Balleine, B. W. (2013). The ventral striato-pallidal pathway mediates the effect of predictive learning on choice between goal-directed actions. *Journal of Neuroscience, 33*(34), 13848-13860.

Manly, J. J., Touradji, P., Tang, M. X., & Stern, Y. (2003). Literacy and memory decline among ethnically diverse elders. *Journal of Clinical and Experimental Neuropsychology, 25*(5), 680-690.

Masten, A. S. (2014). Global perspectives on resilience in children and youth. *Child Development, 85*(1), 6-20.

Mayberg, H. S., Liotti, M., Brannan, S. K., McGinnis, S., Mahurin, R. K., Jerabek, P. A., … Fox, P. T. (1999). Reciprocal limbic-cortical function and negative mood: Converging PET findings in depression and normal sadness. *American Journal of Psychiatry, 156*(5), 675-682.

McCauley, J., Kern, D. E., Kolodner, K., Dill, L., Schroeder, A. F., DeChant, H. K., … Bass, E. B. (1997). Clinical characteristics of women with a history of childhood abuse: unhealed wounds. *JAMA: Journal of the American Medical Association, 277*(17), 1362-1368.doi:10.1001/jama.1997.03540410040028

McEwen, B. S. (2008). Central effects of stress hormones in health and disease: Understanding the protective and damaging effects of stress and stress mediators. *European Journal of Pharmacology, 583*(2-3), 174-185.

McGuire, J. T., & Botvinick, M. M. (2010). Prefrontal cortex, cognitive control, and the registration of decision costs. *Proceedings of the National Academy of Sciences of the United States of America, 107*(17), 7922-7926.

Mickey, B. J., Zhou, Z., Heitzeg, M. M., Heinz, E., Hodgkinson, C. A., Hsu, D. T., … Zubieta, J. K. (2011). Emotion processing, major depression and functional genetic variation of neuropeptide Y. *Archives of General Psychiatry, 68*(2), 158-166.

Middleton, F. A., & Strick, P. L. (2000). Basal ganglia output and cognition: Evidence from anatomical, behavioral, and clinical studies. *Brain and Cognition, 42*(2), 183-200.

Milad, M. R., & Quirk, G. J. (2012). Fear extinction as a model for translational neuroscience: Ten years of progress. *Annual Review of Psychology, 63*, 129-151.

Mink, J. W. (1996). The basal ganglia: Focused selection and inhibition of competing motor programs. *Progress in Neurobiology, 50*(4), 381-425.

Morgan, C. A. 3rd, Rasmusson, A. M., Wang, S., Hoyt, G., Hauger, R. L., & Hazlett, G. (2002). Neuropeptide-Y, cortisol, and subjective distress in humans exposed to acute stress: Replication and extension of previous report. *Biological Psychiatry, 52*(2), 136-142.

Morgan, C. A. 3rd, Wang, S., Southwick, S. M., Rasmusson, A., Hazlett, G., Hauger, R. L., & Charney, D. S. (2000). Plasma neuropeptide-Y concentrations in humans exposed to military survival training. *Biological Psychiatry, 47*(10), 902-909.

Ozbay, F., Fitterling, H., Charney, D., & Southwick, S. (2008). Social support and resilience to stress across the life span: A neurobiologic framework. *Current Psychiatry Reports, 10*(4), 304-310.

Phillips, P. E., Walton, M. E., & Jhou, T. C. (2007). Calculating utility: Preclinical evidence for cost-benefit analysis by mesolimbic dopamine. *Psychopharmacology, 191*(3), 483-495.

Pietrzak, R. H., & Cook, J. M. (2013). Psychological resilience in older U.S. veterans: Results from the national health and resilience in veterans study. *Depression and Anxiety, 30*(5), 432-443.

Plomin, R., Fulker, D. W., Corley, R., & DeFries, J. C. (1997). Nature, nurture, and cognitive development from 1 to 16 years: A parent-offspring adoption study. *Psychological Science, 8*(6), 442-447.

Ramsay, D. S., & Woods, S. C. (2014). Clarifying the roles of homeostasis and allostasis in physiological regulation. *Psychological Review, 121*(2), 225-247.

Reber, J., Feinstein, J. S., O'Doherty, J. P., Liljeholm, M., Adolphs, R., & Tranel, D. (2017). Selective impairment of goal-directed decision-making following lesions to the human ventromedial prefrontal cortex. *Brain, 140*(6), 1743-1756.

Ridderinkhof, K. R., Ullsperger, M., Crone, E. A., & Nieuwenhuis, S. (2004). The role of the medial frontal cortex in cognitive control. *Science, 306*(5695), 443-447.

Ridderinkhof, K. R., van Den Wildenberg, W. P., Segalowitz, S. J., & Carter, C. S. (2004). Neurocognitive mechanisms of cognitive control: The role of prefrontal cortex in action selection, response inhibition, performance monitoring, and reward-based learning. *Brain and Cognition, 56*(2), 129-140.

Rushworth, M. F., Walton, M. E., Kennerley, S. W., & Bannerman, D. M. (2004). Action sets and decisions in the medial frontal cortex. *Trends in Cognitive Sciences, 8*(9), 410-417.

Russo S. J., Murrough J. W., Han M. H., Charney D. S., & Nestler E. J. (2012) Neurobiology of resilience. *Nature Neuroscience, 15*(11), 1475-1484.

Salamone, J. D., Correa, M., Mingote, S., & Weber, S. M. (2003). Nucleus accumbens dopamine and the regulation of effort in food-seeking behavior: Implications for studies of natural motivation, psychiatry, and drug abuse. *Journal of Pharmacology and Experimental Therapeutics, 305*(1), 1-8.

Sanacora, G., Treccani, G., & Popoli, M. (2012). Towards a glutamate hypothesis of depression: An emerging frontier of neuropsychopharmacology for mood disorders. *Neuropharmacology, 62*(1), 63-77.

Schkade, J. K., & McClung, M. (2001). *Occupational adaptation in practice: Concepts and cases.* Thorofare, NJ: SLACK Incorporated.

Schkade, J. K., & Schultz, S. (1992). Occupational adaptation: Toward a holistic approach for contemporary practice, part 1. *American Journal of Occupational Therapy, 46*(9), 829-837.

Schmidt, L., Lebreton, M., Cléry-Melin, M. L., Daunizeau, J., Pessiglione, M. (2012). Neural mechanisms underlying motivation of mental versus physical effort. *Public Library of Science Biology, 10*(2), e1001266. doi:10.1371/journal.pbio.1001266

Schultz, S., & Schkade, J. K. (1992). Occupational adaptation: Toward a holistic approach for contemporary practice, part 2. *American Journal of Occupational Therapy, 46*(10), 917-925.

Schultz, W. (2007). Multiple dopamine functions at different time courses. *Annual Review of Neuroscience, 30*, 259-288.

Seckl, J. R., & Holmes, M. C. (2007). Mechanisms of disease: Glucocorticoids, their placental metabolism and fetal 'programming' of adult pathophysiology. *Nature Reviews Endocrinology, 3*(6), 479-488.

Shonkoff, J., Levitt, P., Bunge, S., Cameron, J., Duncan, G., Fisher, P., & Fox, N. (2015). Supportive relationships and active skill-building strengthen the foundations of resilience. *National Scientific Council on the Developing Child.* Retrieved from https://developingchild.harvard.edu/wp-content/uploads/2015/05/The-Science-of-Resilience.pdf

Simpson, E. H., & Balsam, P. (Eds.). (2016). *Behavioral neuroscience of motivation.* Cham, Switzerland: Springer International.

Sirin, S. R., & Rogers-Sirin, L. (2015). *The educational and mental health needs of Syrian refugee children.* Retrieved from https://www.migrationpolicy.org/research/educational-and-mental-health-needs-syrian-refugee-children

Sørensen, H. J., Mortensen, E. L., Reinisch, J. M., & Mednick, S. A. (2009). Association between prenatal exposure to bacterial infection and risk of schizophrenia. *Schizophrenia Bulletin, 35*(3), 631-637.

Sotres-Bayon, F., & Quirk, G. J. (2010). Prefrontal control of fear: More than just extinction. *Current Opinion in Neurobiology, 20*(2), 231-235.

Sterling, P., & Eyer, J. (1988). Allostasis: A new paradigm to explain arousal pathology. In S. Fisher & J. Reason (Eds.), *Handbook of life stress, cognition and health* (pp. 629-649). Oxford, England: John Wiley & Sons.

Stern, Y. (2009). Cognitive reserve. *Neuropsychologia, 47*(10), 2015-2028.

Turner, L. A., & Johnson, B. (2003). A model of mastery motivation for at-risk preschoolers. *Journal of Educational Psychology, 95*(3), 495-505.

Warden, M. R., Selimbeyoglu, A., Mirzabekov, J. J., Lo, M., Thompson, K. R., Kim, S. Y., … Deisseroth, K. (2012). A prefrontal cortex-brainstem neuronal projection that controls response to behavioural challenge. *Nature, 492*(7429), 428-432.

Whitworth, A. B., & Aichhorn, W. (2005). First-time diagnosis of severe depression: Induced by mefloquine?. *Journal of Clinical Psychopharmacology, 25*(4), 399-400.

Zelazo, P. D., & Carlson, S. M. (2012). Hot and cool executive function in childhood and adolescence: Development and plasticity. *Child Development Perspectives, 6*(4), 354-360.

Zhou, Z., Zhu, G., Hariri, A. R., Enoch, M. A., Scott, D., Sinha, R., … Goldman, D. (2008) Genetic variation in human NPY expression affects stress response and emotion. *Nature, 452*(7190), 997-1001. doi:10.1038/nature06858

Section III

OCCUPATIONAL ADAPTATION IN OCCUPATIONAL THERAPY THEORIES AND MODELS

Lenin C. Grajo, PhD, EdM, OTR/L and Angela K. Boisselle, PhD, OTR, ATP

OVERVIEW

This section highlights a unique perspective to presenting four conceptual models and approaches to occupational therapy intervention—the Occupational Adaptation model, the Model of Human Occupation, the Sensory Processing Model, and the Ecology of Human Performance—by emphasizing how each model defines and applies the construct of occupational adaptation. These conceptual models were chosen to be included in this text because of their explicit framing of the adaptation process as it relates to occupational participation. The importance of the construct of occupational adaptation in occupational therapy's theoretical frameworks is presented through historical and current literature and case examples.

There is a common theme on how each of the four models defines *occupational adaptation*: a process during the person's transaction with the environment. From here, each model elaborates on a unique, truly multidimensional perspective on the construct. Schkade and Schultz's Occupational Adaptation model (Chapter 5) emphasizes the dual nature of the construct—that of a normative and internal human process and as an approach to occupational therapy intervention. Kielhofner's Model of Human Occupation (Chapter 6) focuses on the manner in which occupational adaptation is a process of creating an occupational identity and occupational competence. The Sensory Processing Model (Chapter 7) highlights the adaptive response—the behavioral manifestations of a human's perception of sensory stimuli—which impacts daily occupational participation. Finally, the Ecology of Human Performance (Chapter 8) describes how the adaptation process is critical in understanding a person's task performance range as he or she transacts with properties of the task (occupation) and his or her context.

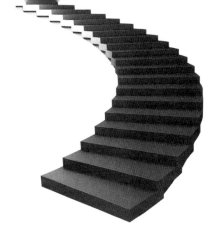

5

Occupational Adaptation as a Normative and Intervention Process

New Perspectives on Schkade and Schultz's Professional Legacy

Lenin C. Grajo, PhD, EdM, OTR/L

OVERVIEW In this chapter, I present a reconceptualization of Schkade and Schultz's Occupational Adaptation (OA) model (1992) as having two core principles:

1. Occupational adaptation is an inherent normative process in humans as occupational beings which may be disrupted by life change, transition, illness or disability; and
2. Occupational adaptation is an intervention process where occupational therapists serve as facilitators to empower within the client the process of change and enable the inherent occupational adaptation process within them.

This chapter aims to present Schkade and Schultz's OA model as a conceptual framework with constructs and language that can be easily applied in daily clinical practice.

Grajo LC, Boisselle AK, eds.
Adaptation Through Occupation:
Multidimensional Perspectives (pp 83-104).
© 2019 SLACK Incorporated.

CHAPTER OBJECTIVES By the end of this chapter, the reader will be able to:

*   Articulate occupational adaptation as an inherent normative process.
*   Articulate how occupational adaptation can be used as an intervention process.
*   Apply constructs of occupational adaptation in daily clinical practice.
*   Develop clinical reasoning and critical thinking strategies to reflect occupational adaptation–guided practice.

GUIDING LEGEND THROUGHOUT THE CHAPTER

*   Occupational Adaptation (OA): capitalized first letters; refers to Schkade and Schultz's model.
*   occupational adaptation: lowercase first letters; refers to the construct of occupational adaptation.

QUESTIONS FOR DISCUSSION AND REFLECTION As the reader explores this chapter, let the following questions guide discussion and reflection:

*   How can I use the language of the OA model in daily practice?
*   What are opportunities and challenges in using the OA model in evaluating and providing intervention for the clients I see in practice?

RATIONALE FOR RECONCEPTUALIZATION

I first published my reconceptualization of Schkade and Schultz's (1992) Occupational Adaptation (OA) model as a chapter in Hinojosa, Kramer, and Royeen's second edition of the *Perspectives on Human Occupation* text (Grajo, 2017). The reconceptualization was precipitated not by the need to change or alter the main principles of the original OA model, but by the need to update and present it in a manner that is more easily applied in daily clinical practice and simplify some of its complex and multitiered constructs. I started that journey by revising the OA process illustration (Schkade & Schultz, 1992; p. 832) to show the holistic and transactive nature of human occupation: the reciprocal and multifaceted relationship between person and environment that emerges during occupational participation, and the entire situational (i.e., defined by what transpires, rather than static) mechanism as the internal process of occupational adaptation (Figure 5-1).

In this chapter, I aim to continue the process of applying the most essential elements of Schkade and Schultz's (1992) OA model based on more current scholarship on clinical applications about the model, including (1) a scoping study of the literature on contemporary applications of the construct of occupational adaptation (see Chapter 1 of this text or Grajo, Boisselle, & DaLomba, 2018); (2) my own clinical research based on applications for children with reading difficulties (Grajo & Candler, 2016a; Grajo & Candler, 2016b); (3) collaborations with clinicians (Grajo & Candler, 2017); and (4) my own interactions and discussions with many students, educators, and clinicians. In this iteration of the reconceptualization, I will also aim to align some of the main constructs of the OA model with the third edition of the Occupational Therapy Practice Framework

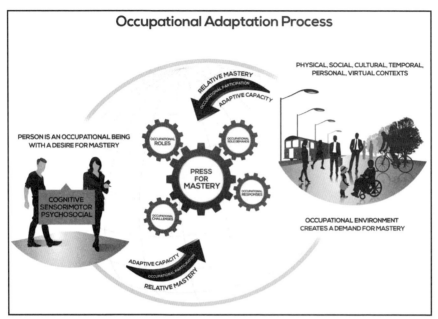

Figure 5-1. A reconceptualization of Schkade and Schultz's Occupational Adaptation process illustration. (Reprinted with permission from Grajo, L. [2017]. Occupational adaptation. In J. Hinojosa, P. Kramer, & C. B. Royeen [Eds.], *Perspectives on human occupation: Theories underlying practice* [2nd ed., pp. 287-311]. Philadelphia, PA: F.A. Davis.)

(Framework III; American Occupational Therapy Association [AOTA], 2014) and the language of the International Classification of Functioning, Disability and Health (ICF; World Health Organization [WHO], 2001). See Table 5-1 for an approximation of OA model concepts with Framework and ICF language.

Although some may think that the legacy of Janette Schkade and Sally Schultz through the OA model may be waning, I actually believe that the work and influence of these two great scholars continue to live on through many scholars who continue to publish work on the construct and the model, and through many of the students they have mentored. As a member of the 2016-2019 Commission on Education of AOTA, we recently revised the Philosophical Base of Occupational Therapy (American Occupational Therapy Association, 2017b) to indicate "participation in occupations is a determinant of health and *leads to adaptation.*" For me, this valuable addition indicates not only the value of the work of many important scholars of the profession, but also the impact of Schkade and Schultz's work on the OA model. Currently, scholarship and practice applications of the model are being published and presented at an increasing rate.

CLARIFYING THE LANGUAGE: STATE AND PROCESS

In the seminal publication of the OA model, Schkade and Schultz (1992) described occupational adaptation as a state and process:

Table 5-1

Occupational Adaptation Model Concepts Juxtaposed With Occupational Therapy Practice Framework and ICF Language		
OA Model Core Constructs	Framework III (American Occupational Therapy Association, 2014)	ICF (World Health Organization, 2002)
Person systems (cognitive, sensorimotor, psychosocial)	Performance skills (motor, process, social interaction skills) Specific client factors (mental, sensory, neuromusculoskeletal, and movement functions)	Body functions and body structures
Occupational environment	Contexts (cultural, personal temporal, virtual) Environments (physical and social)	Environmental factors
Occupational participation	Participation	Participation
Occupation	Occupations (activities of daily living, instrumental activities of daily living, rest and sleep, education, work, play, leisure, social participation)	Activity
Press for mastery		
Occupational roles	Roles	
Occupational challenges		
Role demands and expectations	Occupational demands	
Occupational responses		

Adapted from American Occupational Therapy Association. (2014). Occupational therapy practice framework: Domain and process (3rd ed.). *American Journal of Occupational Therapy, 68,* S1-S48. doi:10.5014/ajot.2014.682006 and World Health Organization. (2001). *International Classification of Functioning, Disability and Health (ICF).* Geneva, Switzerland: World Health Organization.

Occupational adaptation (state) is a state of competency in occupational functioning toward which humans aspire.

Occupational adaptation (process) is the process through which the person and the occupational environment interact when the person is faced with occupational challenges calling for an occupational response reflecting an experience of relative mastery. (p. 831)

This state and process aspect of occupational adaptation is most confusing to many who aim to study and use the model. Do you evaluate occupational adaptation as state, process, or both? Which comes first, the process or the state? Can there be a state without the process and vice versa? How do we know if what the scholar is intending to describe is occupational adaptation as a state or as a process?

When my colleagues, Drs. Angie Boisselle and Elaina DaLomba, and I did the scoping study on the construct of occupational adaptation (see Chapter 1), we faced a similar dilemma of having to parse out the two terms when coding the studies and having to clearly explain the construct to scholars and reviewers, and eventually to the audience of the manuscript. In the scoping study, we assert that scholars and practitioners must clearly articulate and explain how they are using the construct of occupational adaptation (Grajo et al., 2018) to advance the knowledge about the construct.

For purposes of language and clarification, here I propose that occupational adaptation is an inherent process within the person, following Schkade and Schultz's definition of occupational adaptation as a process (1992). Occupational adaptation is also an intervention model, an approach to occupational therapy assessment and intervention (following Schultz & Schkade's [1992] assertion that it is also a practice model). When a state of competency has been achieved during the iterative process of occupational adaptation and/or as a result of occupational therapy service provision, a client or the person may achieve a state *occupational adaptiveness*.

CORE PRINCIPLE 1: OCCUPATIONAL ADAPTATION IS AN INTERNAL NORMATIVE PROCESS

In this chapter, I will use two case stories to contextualize the different constructs and applications of the OA model. Schkade and Schultz (2003) highlighted three main constructs in the OA model (which are referred to as constants in various texts): the *person*, the *occupational environment*, and the *press for mastery*. The press for mastery is the situational construct that emerges when the person and the environment transact during occupational participation. In this reconceptualization, I assert that *occupational participation* is another core constant, central to the OA model. Let us begin understanding these four constructs and the principle of OA as a normative process using the case study below. Refer back to Figure 5-1 for the illustration of the internal OA process.

> **CASE STUDY: JENNIFER** Jennifer is a special education teacher who recently got married to her partner. After several years of contemplating about her readiness for graduate school, Jennifer decided to enroll for a Doctor of Education program offered online. She is now needing to balance many different roles, such as being a partner, a full-time teacher, and a part-time graduate student taking six credits of course work per semester.

OA Construct: The Person

The person is an occupational being who desires to master occupations through transactions with the environment (Grajo, 2017). The person comprises three person systems that enable the person to perform and participate in occupations: cognitive, sensorimotor, and psychosocial systems (Schkade & Schultz, 2003). These person systems can be understood parallel to, but not directly in relation to, the Framework's *performance skills* (motor, process, and social interaction skills) and *body functions* (mental functions, sensory functions, neuromusculoskeletal functions) within *client factors* (American Occupational Therapy Association, 2014), and the ICF's *body functions* and *body structures* (World Health Organization, 2001). The person's sense of self and identity is shaped by the occupations that he or she chooses to participate in, in fulfillment of many important occupational roles, routines, rituals, and habits (*performance patterns* in the Framework; American Occupational Therapy Association, 2014). Inherent to the person is this *desire to master occupations* and to navigate his or her occupational environment with mastery and competence.

In the case of Jennifer, we can assume that she has a desire to master different occupations related to her roles of being a teacher, a partner, and a graduate student. For example, as a teacher, we can assume that she wants to master occupations such as preparing teaching plans and participating in reviewing and revising Individualized Educational Plans (IEPs) for her students. These occupations and the desire to master them will shape how she will transact with her occupational environments.

OA Construct: The Occupational Environment

The occupational environment includes settings and contexts that influence occupational performance and participation. In Framework III terms, the occupational environment comprises *contexts* (cultural, personal, temporal, virtual) and *environments* (physical and social) that are interrelated conditions within and surrounding the client and in which daily life occupations occur (American Occupational Therapy Association, 2014). In ICF language, the occupational environment may refer to *environmental factors* that make up the physical, social, and attitudinal environment in which people live and conduct their lives (World Health Organization, 2001). Inherent to the occupational environment is a *demand for mastery* from the person.

In the case of Jennifer, let us consider one occupational environment: the school setting where she works as a special education teacher. This occupational environment may demand from Jennifer that she is always on time and present at work; able to meet students who need special education instruction; able to meet and discuss with parents, school psychologists, and therapists about students; and able to meet deadlines.

OA Construct: Occupational Participation

Perhaps central to the OA model and the profession of occupational therapy is occupational participation. According to Schkade and Schultz (2003), occupations have three important properties: they (1) require active engagement, (2) have meaning to the individual, and (3) are goal oriented (Grajo, 2017; from the original Schkade & Schultz

[1992] model, the third property of occupation is that it creates a tangible or intangible product as a result of a process). *Occupations*, according to the Framework III, include activities of daily living, instrumental activities of daily living, rest and sleep, education, work, play, leisure, and social participation (American Occupational Therapy Association, 2014). The overarching theme of the domain and process of occupational therapy is "achieving health, well-being, and participation in life through engagement in occupation" (p. S4). In the ICF, *activity* (execution of a task by the individual) and *participation* (involvement in a life situation) (World Health Organization, 2001) are corresponding terms to occupational participation in the model. According to Schkade and Schultz (2003), occupations are the mechanisms for occupational adaptation as an internal process to manifest.

OA Construct: Press for Mastery

The press for mastery is the transaction between the person (with the desire for mastery) and the occupational environment (with the demand for mastery). This transaction is manifested during participation in occupations. Several processes within the press for mastery are simultaneously or concurrently activated when a person perceives a demand for mastery from the environment and calibrates this demand with his or her level of desire for mastery and level of abilities based on the person systems (cognitive, sensorimotor, psychosocial). Collectively, these processes comprise the press for mastery:

- **Occupational roles.** According to the Framework III, roles are sets of behaviors expected by society and shaped by culture and context that maybe further conceptualized and defined by the client (American Occupational Therapy Association, 2014, p. S27).

- **Occupational challenges**. As the person calibrates the demand for mastery from the environment, his or her abilities (based on person systems), level of motivation (desire for mastery), and perceived or observable level of occupational challenge may become evident. Some occupational challenges are easily surmountable (when demand for mastery, desire for mastery, and person system abilities are of equal levels or capacities), whereas some may lead the client to a level of occupational dysadaptation (when desire for mastery is high, demand for mastery is high or low, and person system abilities are low). See Figure 5-2 for an illustration of potential calibrations of the press for mastery. Indirectly, occupational challenges can be similar to *occupational demands* in the Framework III because, based on the person's needs and contexts, the demands of the occupation can be seen as barriers or supports to occupational participation (American Occupational Therapy Association, 2014, p. S32) and include the relevance and importance of the occupation to the person and other physical and social demands, resources, actions, and skills required of the person.

- **Role demands or expectations.** When an occupational challenge is perceived or foreseen, the person once again calibrates his or her desire for mastery, demand for mastery from the environment, person system abilities, and occupational roles and kinds of occupations expected to be performed as part of these roles. This forms internal role demands (perceived by the person) or external role demands (asserted by the occupational environment) or both.

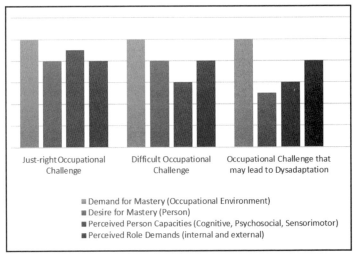

Figure 5-2. Different levels of occupational challenges that activate the normative occupational adaptation process in humans as occupational beings.

- **Occupational responses.** As the person calibrates the occupational challenges, roles, and role demands and identifies a way to plan and produce a manner of responding to participate in occupations, the person configures an adaptation gestalt. The *adaptation gestalt* allows the person to determine whether to choose from a previously used occupational response that successfully overcame or managed the occupational challenge, create a new occupational response when an old one is not available or useful, or modify a previously used response.

The Adaptation Gestalt

When describing the press for mastery components, I mentioned several times that the person will need to calibrate his or her person system abilities, his or her desire for mastery, and the occupational environment's demand for mastery. To calibrate the person system abilities to enable the person to develop a plan of response on how to participate and perform occupations and overcome occupational challenges, the person will need to configure his or her adaptation gestalt. The adaptation gestalt is a manner of configuring the amount and level of cognitive, sensorimotor, and psychosocial capacities to determine how to perform an occupation with a level of mastery and competence (Schkade & Schultz, 1992). Certain occupations and occupational challenges will require more cognitive capacities than psychosocial and sensorimotor abilities (e.g., solving a crossword puzzle). Some occupations and challenges will require a slightly more set of psychosocial abilities (e.g., interacting and socializing at a party). The adaptation gestalt can be visualized as a pie chart (Schultz & Schkade, 1997). This can be a helpful tool for a person to analyze how to properly configure his or her abilities and the demands of the occupation. In the pie chart visual analogy, the person system that is required more to perform an occupation is said to have a bigger configuration in the adaptation gestalt. Likewise, when a person system is deficient (e.g., an older adult having memory decline, and therefore a deficient cognitive system), that person system is overriding the adaptation gestalt (Grajo, 2017).

Adaptive and Dysadaptive Responses

Schkade and Schultz's model (1992) describes a multilayered *adaptive response mechanism*. Here, I simplify the approach to understanding this complex mechanism as part of the occupational response process. In the original process illustration of the OA model (Schkade & Schultz, 1992, p. 832), this adaptive response mechanism is identified as a process that happens within the person stemming out of the press for mastery. In this reconceptualization, I argue that the adaptive mechanism is still part of the situational and transactional aspect of the occupational adaptation process, within the press for mastery. As the person participates in occupations within the occupational environment, the person performs an ongoing trial-and-error process of calibrating roles, role demands, and occupational challenges and identifying occupational responses that may create mastery and competence in occupation. This trial-and-error process may include one or more occupational responses, evaluating whether the response(s) achieves mastery and competence and overcomes the occupational challenge, and modifying and integrating responses to determine how best to solve occupational challenges and participate in occupations masterfully in the future. Some responses may be *adaptive*, or those that overcome or effectively manage the occupational challenges and promote mastery and competence in the occupation, and some responses may be *dysadaptive*, a term coined within the model (Schkade & Schultz, 1992) to describe when responses do not overcome the occupational challenge. As a person participates in occupations and encounters occupational challenges, he or she may use a series and combination of adaptive and dysadaptive responses in an ongoing and iterative process.

To apply the processes within the press for mastery and the concept of the adaptation gestalt, let's go back to the case of Jennifer. See Figure 5-3 for a visual analysis of the press for mastery. This time, let's analyze Jennifer's occupational role as a graduate student. Jennifer wants to make sure that she is able to maximize all learning opportunities and earn strong grades for graduate school (desire for mastery). Her occupational environments (home shared with partner, special education school, graduate school) all want Jennifer to be able to juggle her various roles and tasks extremely well (demand for mastery). On top of her role as a graduate student, she knows she has multiple other roles, such as being a loving partner, an excellent special education teacher, and an outstanding graduate student (occupational roles). She knows that she needs to manage her time extremely well, balance responsibilities, and devote appropriate time and energy to fulfill all her existing and new roles (internal and external role demands). To do this, Jennifer will need to configure her adaptation gestalt to allow her to identify whether to use her existing time management tools (existing occupational response) or to develop or modify new ways of managing her time based on trial and error or advice from her graduate school mentors and peers (new and modified responses). For example, to cope with stress, Jennifer decided that she will regularly participate in yoga classes (adaptive response). However, sometimes, when she is exhausted and overwhelmed with graduate school assignments, she will skip yoga and start to binge watch and stream some television shows online (potentially dysadaptive response).

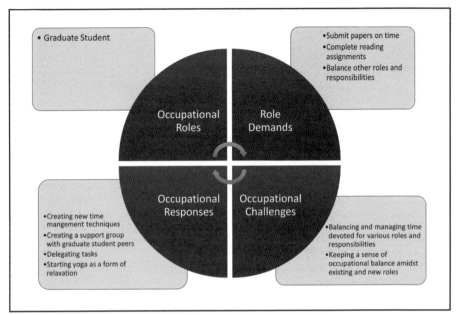

Figure 5-3. Configuring the press for mastery: Jennifer's case.

The entire iterative process of calibration, trial and error, and participating in occupations while balancing internal and external demands, levels of desire, and demand for mastery is the core of the occupational adaptation process as a normative, internal process.

Measuring Occupational Adaptation

As occupational beings, we juggle many occupational roles and responsibilities each day. We navigate through multiple occupational challenges, sometimes one at a time, sometimes many at a time. We set expectations for ourselves, and our occupational environments set expectations that become various levels of perceived role demands. These ways of daily life require us to be occupationally adaptive (state). Many times, we respond to challenges using tools and strategies we have used before. Sometimes we fail at challenges and move on. There are also times when we become stuck when faced with very difficult occupational challenges, and these moments are states of *occupational dysadaptation*. How do we know if we are in this state? Two terms have been used in the OA model to describe how to assess whether the normative process of occupational adaptation is working and when a state of occupational adaptiveness is achieved: *relative mastery* and *adaptive capacity*.

Relative Mastery

I have adapted the definition of relative mastery (Grajo, 2017, p. 297) from Schkade and McClung (2001) to have three components:

1. *Effective participation* in occupations is assessed based on how well people achieve their set goals of occupational engagement and participation.
2. *Efficiency* is a person's good and appropriate use of available personal resources and resources in the occupational environment (e.g., time, energy, task objects and materials, social supports).
3. *Satisfaction* is the extent to which people are content with their occupational performance and the congruence between occupational participation and performance expectations. Satisfaction is measured based on self and satisfaction of important others.

Adaptive Capacity

Adaptive capacity is the person's ability to perceive the need to change, modify, or refine a variety of responses to occupational challenges in the environment (Schkade & Schultz, 2003). I like using the analogy of "tools in a toolbox" (Grajo, 2017) when describing adaptive capacity. Does the person have enough tools in his or her toolbox to respond to the occupational challenge? When there are existing tools, is the person able to choose appropriate tools or strategies to respond to the challenge? If there are no previously used tools or strategies, is the person able to creatively come up with strategies and tools? Is he or she able to adapt or modify previously used tools and strategies to help with this occupational challenge?

Let us apply the assessment of occupational adaptation in the case of Jennifer. See Figure 5-4 for a set of questions that can be asked to assess her relative mastery and adaptive capacity. Assume that Jennifer has started to experience increased levels of stress as a new graduate student who is also juggling work responsibilities and preparing for her wedding and new life with her fiancé. She is able to submit papers on time; however, she feels that she is always beating the deadline, exhausted, and feeling behind in completing her weekly course readings. To assess her relative mastery, it is important to inquire about her perceived levels of effectiveness in achieving goals related to graduate school studies; her level of efficiency or her use of time, resources, tools, and materials to achieve goals; and her level of satisfaction, and that of important others (fiancé), after completion of the goal or occupation. When assessing her adaptive capacity, it is important to first inquire about her insight on what her occupational challenges are and how she is handling these occupational challenges. Next, we can inquire about the tools and strategies she has used in previous situations or previous similar challenges. It is then critical to assess her insight on whether using these tools might work for the present challenge or whether new or modified tools may need to be created based on previous experiences. As with life, a person's occupational adaptiveness will go through a series of trial and error. Is the person able to get him- or herself "unstuck" when faced with the occupational challenge? Is the person demonstrating relative mastery and use of adaptive capacities when faced with several occupational challenges? Is the person in a constant state of being "stuck" when performing daily occupations? Is the person going through a state of life transition or a state of illness or disability? How is this transition or state of illness or disability impact-

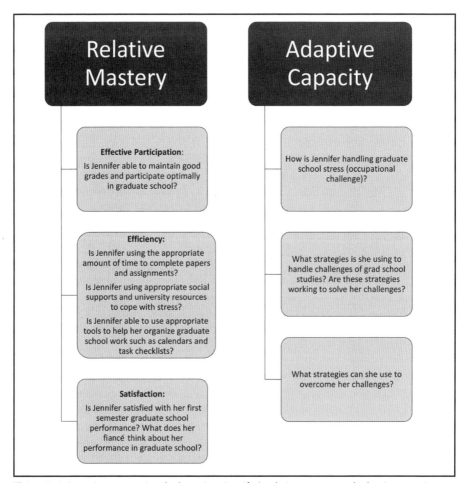

Figure 5-4. Assessing occupational adaptation: Jennifer's relative mastery and adaptive capacity.

ing the person's occupational adaptation process? When a person goes through a state of life transition and/or a state of disability and his or her state and process of occupational adaptation is impacted so that the person is unable to perform daily occupations and participate in life with relative mastery and adaptive capacity, an occupational therapy practitioner may be able to support the person.

CORE PRINCIPLE 2: OCCUPATIONAL ADAPTATION AS AN INTERVENTION PROCESS

When a person is unable to live life meaningfully and/or participate in occupations optimally, the person's occupational adaptation process may be negatively impacted. A state of occupational dysadaptation may be most evident during a time of major life transition, or as a result of atypical growth and development, state of illness, or disability (Grajo, 2017). Occupational dysadaptation may include the inability to perform occupational roles, difficulty participating in occupations or completing tasks related to occupations, difficulty overcoming occupational challenges, being overwhelmed by role demands and responsibilities, and/or the inability to use appropriate tools or strategies to overcome occupational or task performance breakdown. Some people are able to resolve temporary states of occupational dysadaptation, whereas others remain, or foresee remaining, in this state for a prolonged period of time. In this case, occupational therapy can support this person and be guided by the OA model. I will use the following case of Olenna to illustrate elements of OA-guided intervention.

> CASE STUDY: OLENNA Olenna is a pharmacist who is married and has adult kids. She has recently been diagnosed with stage 3 breast cancer, had a total mastectomy after neoadjuvant chemotherapy, received radiation treatments, and has started receiving monthly treatments of chemotherapy. She has taken a leave at the pharmacy and is feeling depressed and withdrawn. She has a supportive husband and children. Her surgery has caused some bilateral arm movement limitations that triggered lymphedema and some balance issues that have hindered her from being able to play with her young grandchildren, cook meals for herself and her husband, and perform some daily occupations, such as dressing. She is also experiencing cognitive deficits, such as mild memory loss and some occasional disorientation. She was referred to occupational therapy for evaluation and treatment. When asked about her important roles she wants to prioritize, she replied, "I want to be able to care for myself and my husband again and play with my grandchildren. My children and grandchildren's weekly visits and my making brunch for them on Sundays are the most important thing for me. I hope I will also be able to get back to work soon."

OA-guided intervention is not a protocol or a series of action steps to do or to take. The OA model is a conceptual model. Conceptual practice models offer theories that serve as a way of thinking about and doing practice. They generate practice resources and guide research that supports evidence-based practice, and they are critically important in growing the profession and individual practice (Kielhofner, 2009). In my reconceptualization of occupational adaptation as a framework for occupational therapy intervention (Grajo, 2017), I highlighted some key principles or guidelines that are essential in OA-guided intervention based on intervention principles stated by Schultz (2014). These guidelines are a manner of thinking about doing occupational therapy assessment and intervention rather than specific steps that the therapist must do. According to Schultz and Schkade (1997), occupational adaptation is not a collection of techniques but a way of directing the therapist's thinking about intervention in the person's internal adaptation process. Therefore, these guidelines are open to ways of being modified to best suit the demands of the occupational therapist's practice setting, state- or country-defined practice guidelines, and models of service payment. There is also criticism that many occupation-based models developed in the United States are developed with a Western mindset and may not be as culturally relevant to patients and practitioners from other countries. OA as a conceptual model is based on widely accepted constructs deeply rooted in the history of the profession, which I highlighted in the first reconceptualization

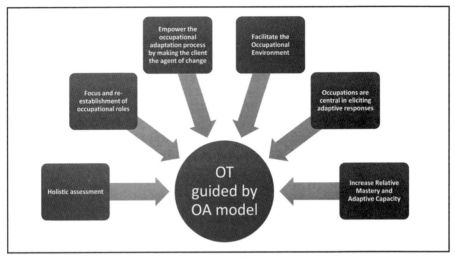

Figure 5-5. Intervention guidelines using the OA model.

(Grajo, 2017, p. 288), and therefore should make the model easy to adapt for culturally relevant practice in any setting. Some of these historical underpinnings included use of occupation to facilitate adaptation (Meyer, 1922/1977); man's need to master the environment (Reilly, 1962); occupation as a way to achieve competency, mastery, and motivation (Florey, 1969; Llorens, 1970; White, 1959); the importance of self-initiated occupation (Yerxa, 1967); and different perspectives and definitions of adaptation, competence, and resilience as a result of doing, active involvement, and choice (Fidler, 1981; Fidler & Fidler, 1978; Fine, 1991; Kielhofner, 1977; King, 1978; Kleinman & Buckley, 1982; Nelson, 1988). Additionally, the construct and the model have been used and applied in research in other countries (Nayar & Stanley, 2014; Soeker, 2011) (see Chapters 1 and 10).

In this chapter, I expand Schultz's (2014) occupational adaptation intervention guidelines to have six essential elements (Figure 5-5):

1. Use of holistic assessment
2. Focus and reestablishment of occupational roles
3. Use of occupations is central in eliciting adaptive responses
4. Empower the occupational adaptation process by making the client the agent of change
5. Facilitate the occupational environment
6. Increase relative mastery and adaptive capacity

Element 1: Use of Holistic Assessment

The OA model does not prescribe the use of any specific assessments. However, the OA model encourages the use of a combination of standardized and nonstandardized assessments (Royeen, Grajo, & Luebben, 2014). Schultz (2014) emphasized that assessments should not only measure static outcomes but also assess the impact of the intervention on the client's engagement and personally meaningful life roles. Assessments used in the evaluation process need to provide a clear and holistic picture of the client's occupational profile. Norm-referenced tools can be used in combination with patient report–type tools and observation of occupational performance and participation. An analysis of natural contexts of occupational participation can be done through questionnaires and interviews if observations and assessment of the actual contexts of performance cannot be done. An analysis of the client's relative mastery and adaptive capacity can be done as part of formulating an occupational profile.

Some questions to assess relative mastery may include the following (Grajo, 2017, p. 298):

- **Effectiveness**: Can you complete the task successfully? How much assistance do you need? Which steps of the task did you find difficult?
- **Efficiency**: Describe the amount of time you need to complete the task/activity. Do you require any tools to complete the task? Do you have access to these tools and resources? Describe the amount of energy or effort you require to complete the task.
- **Satisfaction**: How do you feel about the quality of your task performance/completion? How do important others (spouse/children/peers/employers) feel about your task performance/completion?

Some questions to assess adaptive capacity may include the following (Grajo, 2017, p. 298):

- When you feel like you are having difficulty completing the task, what do you do?
- What tools or strategies do you use when you experience challenges completing the task?
- Do you think the tools that you use work? What do you do if your strategy doesn't work this time?
- How do you cope with frustration when faced with a challenge that's hard to overcome?

Now let us apply this element in Olenna's case. The occupational therapy practitioner guided by occupational adaptation will begin by creating an occupational profile. AOTA's Occupational Profile template (2017a) can be a useful tool to begin this process, while also asking questions related to the client's occupational adaptiveness (relative mastery and adaptive capacity). The occupational therapist might use a variety of functional and standardized tools to assess upper extremity functioning, level of edema, functional cognition, strength and endurance, and sensory-perceptual tests to assess factors that may impact occupational performance. The therapist can use patient goal-setting tools such as the Canadian Occupational Performance Measure (Law et al., 2005) to set occupational goals that are relevant to the client.

Element 2: Focus and Reestablishment of Occupational Roles

The OA model supports a client-centered, role-focused approach rather than development of performance skills. OA-guided interventions focus on identifying roles that are essential to the client (Schkade & Schultz, 2003) and increasing the client's occupational adaptiveness to facilitate participation in occupations and fulfill these essential occupational roles (Grajo, 2017). Life roles provide the context for expressing our competence in occupational functioning (Schkade & McClung, 2001). Another critical notion of the model is that the occupational therapist must focus on one role at a time (Schkade & Schultz, 2003). During a major life transition or state of disability, the client may be experiencing a major disruption of the occupational adaptation process. Habits and routines may be altered. The person's understanding of his or her occupational identity may have changed and may be continuously changing. Valued occupational roles and responsibilities may shift and change. It is essential to the OA-guided therapist to facilitate the client's prioritization of meaningful roles and start empowering the client's occupational adaptation process (see Element 3 for more details) through a series of calibrated tasks and occupations that will stimulate adaptive responses (see Element 5 for more details).

This element of OA-guided intervention is very apparent in Olenna's case. She articulated that she wants to be able to participate in occupations related to her care of self and her husband; participate in caring for, playing with, and preparing meals for her children and grandchildren; and eventually go back to her job. Her important roles are being an independent person, wife, grandmother, mother, and pharmacist. The occupational therapist will ask Olenna to prioritize one role at a time and work on reestablishing her ability to participate in occupations related to this important role.

Element 3: Empower the Occupational Adaptation Process by Making the Client the Agent of Change

Elizabeth Yerxa's body of work is one of the many historical underpinnings of Schkade and Schultz's model (Schultz & Schkade, 1997). In her 1966 Slagle Lecture, Yerxa described that "authentic occupational therapy is based upon a commitment to the client's realization of his own particular meaning" (1967, p. 8). She added that "choice" and "self-initiated purposeful activity" are what make our profession unique (p. 8). These concepts are central to OA-guided intervention. In an editorial on occupation, occupational adaptation, and client-centeredness, Grajo and Cruz (2017) asserted that, oftentimes, with the pressure of health care reimbursement policies and workplace protocols, occupational therapy practitioners often neglect the value of choice and self-initiated goals and occupations. Critical in OA-guided intervention is making the client the agent of change in the therapeutic process. This can be facilitated by allowing the client and his or her family the freedom and choice to set meaningful goals throughout the intervention, choose occupations to work on, and make critical decisions about progression of therapy. When the client's cognitive abilities or levels of insight and awareness may hinder full self-initiation of goals and identification of occupations, the occupational therapist can provide choices based on information gathered from the client's evaluation and occupational profile. The therapist can work collaboratively with the family and the health care team to ensure that choices made best represent what the client and family think is best rather than what the therapist thinks is best for the client. When the client is empowered as an agent of change, he or she is better able to calibrate his or her desire to master the occupation and anticipate the demands for mastery by the occupational environment, and the occupational adaptation process is also then empowered. In using this element of the intervention, the OA-guided therapist uses his or her critical and clinical reasoning skills and clinical experience to carefully and strategically use probing and facilitated questions rather than telling the client what needs to be done.

In Olenna's case, because of reported feelings of depression and withdrawal, the occupational therapist can start therapy sessions by asking about occupations and functional tasks that she would like to work on for that day. Goals related to upper extremity function and reduction of edema can be embedded within tasks and occupations that she finds interesting for the day. By focusing on occupational roles, such as being a wife or grandmother, the occupational therapist can provide choices of occupations that Olenna might be interested in if she continues to be withdrawn and lacks initiative to participate in the therapy. For example, the therapist can ask, "Would you like to work on frosting and decorating cookies? Maybe we can save some of them and put them in nice boxes for you to give to your grandchildren when they visit you?" or rephrase this with a broader question of, "Is there anything you would like to do today where we can make you use your arms and hands and create something you can give to your grandchildren when they visit you? You can tell them you worked hard on this during your therapy and I am sure they will enjoy it!"

Element 4: Occupations Are Central in Eliciting Adaptive Responses

Occupations are central in facilitating adaptive responses from the client. When a client feels stuck and in a constant or intermittent state of occupational dysadaptation, the therapist can use occupations to facilitate the client getting him- or herself "unstuck." Schultz and Schkade (1992) described two components of OA-guided intervention: occupational readiness and occupational activities. *Occupational readiness* aims to prepare the person systems (cognitive, sensorimotor, and psychosocial capacities) to engage in occupations (Schkade & McClung, 2001). Occupational readiness can be described as preparatory activities or performance skill-building approaches. In the case of Olenna, the therapist may use a variety of decongestive therapies, such as exercise, compression garments, or manual lymph drainage, to facilitate use of her upper extremities in preparation for occupations. *Occupational activities* simulate or replicate tasks of the meaningful occupational role (Schkade & McClung, 2001). Occupational activities may use contrived contexts or tools, especially when clients are limited by the contexts of where occupational therapy services are provided (e.g., hospital bed or room, clinic kitchen or activities of daily living room). In the case of Olenna, the therapist may invite her to do some light meal preparation activities in the kitchen space using tools and materials that the therapist has prepared.

It is essential in any occupational therapy intervention to facilitate the use of natural contexts. The therapist guided by OA must try to move away from occupational readiness and use of simulated tasks as quickly as possible and encourage use of materials, tools, and environments where natural occupational participation occurs. In the case of Olenna, it may be impossible to do light meal preparation in her home kitchen, but the therapist can encourage use of ingredients that she likes, ask her to bring her apron or oven mitts from home, and approximate the size and weight of bowls and pans that she uses. The therapist is skilled in occupational analysis (American Occupational Therapy Association, 2014) and will carefully adjust the level of occupational challenge so that adaptive responses are elicited from the client. For example, the therapist may ask Olenna to remember to carry an increasing number of household items and ingredients from the cupboard to the kitchen counter. This may elicit tools and strategies that Olenna will need to use to remember the list of household items and to transport the items with as little energy expenditure and time as possible.

Element 5: Facilitate the Occupational Environment

Similar to the skillful use of occupations to facilitate and elicit adaptive responses, the occupational therapist also facilitates the occupational environment to empower the occupational adaption process of the client. The therapist may modify the physical environment by helping the client identify barriers and supporters of occupational participation and problem solve with the client how the physical environment can be modified to enhance participation. The therapist may also facilitate the use of social contexts (e.g., family members, friends) to create role demands and expectations and encourage the client to participate more in the occupations and the therapy process. Similar to the essential element of use of occupations, the therapist must encourage the use of natural environments and social contexts during intervention. In the case of Olenna, the therapist might encourage her husband or, if possible, her grandchildren to participate and use co-occupations (mutually engaged-in occupations) such as playing board games or making dessert. The therapist can also problem solve with Olenna on how to modify and make adaptations to kitchen tools that she uses at home so she is able to hold and use them.

Element 6: Increase Relative Mastery and Adaptive Capacity

Using the different elements of OA-guided intervention, the occupational therapist will aim to increase the client's occupational adaptiveness by increasing relative mastery and adaptive capacity. The following are some key questions to determine whether a state of occupational adaptiveness is restored or being facilitated:

- Is the client able to achieve occupational goals (effective participation)?
- Is the client able to participate in occupations within an acceptable amount of time, using appropriate energy and resources (efficiency)?
- Is the client and his or her important others satisfied with the occupational performance (satisfaction)?
- Is the client able to apply and use a variety of tools and strategies to overcome occupational challenges (adaptive capacity)?
- Is the client able to independently perform and identify occupations that he or she wants to engage in despite foreseen occupational challenges (initiation)?
- Is the client able to use existing tools/strategies in similar or other occupational challenges (transfer of learning)?

- Is the client able to come up with new tools/strategies or modify old strategies to solve similar or new occupational challenges (generalization)?

The OA-guided occupational therapist will use clinical reasoning, critical thinking abilities, and creativity to skillfully use and modify these six elements of intervention to make sure that services provided are culturally relevant, are centered on the needs of the client, and empower the occupational adaptation process of the client.

INSIGHTS FROM A CLINICAL APPLICATION OF OCCUPATIONAL ADAPTATION

Throughout this book, several chapters present research on and clinical applications of the OA model to provide insights on how it can be applied in clinical practice. I want to highlight in this chapter some excerpts from my own clinical research and some of the perspectives of clinicians who have discovered the power of Schkade and Schultz's OA model. In 2015, I conducted a pilot Community of Practice (Wenger, 2000) that included 12 pediatric occupational therapists working in schools, private practice, and hospital settings who wanted to learn how therapists can better support children with literacy challenges. The Community of Practice is based on training occupational therapists on how to apply the Occupation and Participation Approach to Reading Intervention (OPARI; Grajo & Candler, 2016b), an OA-guided approach to supporting children with reading difficulties. During a 7-month immersive process, participants learned about the OA model and how to use it in practice. The following are some excerpts from two publications about the Community of Practice process and clinicians' insights on the use of the OA model and its impact on their practice:

> The community of practice has been a sort of gentle "poke in my side" to make me remember many of the basics of [occupational therapy] that I learned in school: theory, participation, and true occupation (Grajo & Candler, 2017, p. 8).

> I definitely used to see my role as "fixer" and targeting skills with the use of activities that emphasized these specific skills. Now I find that I facilitate the betterment of the child and parent/caregiver, through participation from the moment the assessment begins (Grajo & Candler, 2017, p. 7).

> Ever diligent, I labored to improve my client's fine motor, visual motor, and school-related skills, aiming for their optimum performance. But I had not known or embraced Occupational Adaptation Theory—that push for client-generated activities that would magnify meaning and activate the client to become his or her own agent of change…. Here's the thing: I have always employed creative and fun activities in my practice, but I did not tailor those activities to each child's most motivating interests…. However, as I employed more client-generated choices, I witnessed more vigorous responses to intervention, as children took over my sessions…. Student-generated strategies brought forth hilarity and magic (Grajo et al., 2016, p. 12).

Although occupational adaptation is a complex, often very abstract phenomenon (Grajo, Boisselle, & DaLomba, 2018), the OA model can be easily applied to guide daily practice and better understand our clients as occupational beings. Many clinicians who get to use the OA model in their practice and research find how the understanding of occupational adaptation as a normative process makes it easier for them to appreciate and shift the way they do occupational therapy in their practice settings.

ADVANCING THE KNOWLEDGE ON OCCUPATIONAL ADAPTATION

This chapter is an ongoing effort to evolve and continue to grow this great conceptual model that Drs. Janette Schkade and Sally Schultz have contributed to the body of knowledge and science of occupational therapy. Having been mentored by Sally Schultz, I am greatly indebted to the wisdom she shared with me and countless graduate students at Texas Woman's University. Most importantly, I am so grateful for her inspiration and her trust in me to continue writing about the OA model.

Occupational adaptation is a culturally relevant construct and model. Occupational adaptation is a process that happens within the person that allows him or her to respond with mastery and competence in the occupational environment during performance and participation in occupations. OA is also an intervention model to guide occupational therapy practitioners in their manner of thinking and working with the client, to empower the occupational adaptation process and facilitate the client as an agent of change, and to enable him or her to live life optimally. Schkade and Schultz (in Schkade & Mc-Clung, 2001) assert that the occupational therapist guided by this model must not aim to fix everything in the client. Like one of the clinicians in my community of practice stated, we must not be "fixers" for our clients. Use Schkade and Schultz's OA model and empower clients to overcome their daily challenges and gain a sense of mastery and competence in their daily occupational roles.

SUMMARY AND IMPLICATIONS

- Occupational adaptation is an internal normative process that describes the transaction between the person and the environment during participation in daily occupations. This process is iterative and a manner of calibrating occupational roles, role demands, and occupational challenges so the person is able to respond adaptively to these challenges.
- Occupational Adaptation is a conceptual model for intervention. It describes how the occupational therapist is a facilitator within the therapeutic context and the client is the agent of change in the process. The therapist guided by this intervention model provides holistic assessment, focuses on occupational roles, and empowers the client as an agent of change by use of occupations and facilitating the environment, to increase the client's relative mastery and adaptive capacity.

- Occupational adaptiveness is a state we aim to achieve for ourselves and for our clients. A person who is occupationally adaptive is able to participate and perform occupations with relative mastery and uses his or her adaptive capacities to overcome occupational challenges. All humans go through states of occupational adaptation and dysadaptation. A constant state of occupational dysadaptiveness may necessitate occupational therapy services.

REFERENCES

American Occupational Therapy Association. (2014). Occupational therapy practice framework: Domain and process (3rd ed.). *American Journal of Occupational Therapy, 68*(Suppl. 1), S1-S48. doi:10.5014/ajot.2014.682006

American Occupational Therapy Association. (2017a). AOTA occupational profile template. Retrieved from https://www.aota.org/-/media/Corporate/Files/Practice/Manage/Documentation/AOTA-Occupational-Profile-Template.pdf

American Occupational Therapy Association. (2017b). Philosophical base of occupational therapy. *American Journal of Occupational Therapy, 71*(Suppl. 2), 7112410045. doi:10.5014/ajot.2017.716S06

Fidler, G. S. (1981). From crafts to competence. *American Journal of Occupational Therapy, 35*(9), 567-573. doi:10.5014/ajot.35.9.567

Fidler, G. S., & Fidler, J. W. (1978). Doing and becoming: Purposeful action and self-actualization. *American Journal of Occupational Therapy, 32*(5), 305-310.

Fine, S. B. (1991). Resilience and human adaptability: Who rises above adversity? *American Journal of Occupational Therapy, 45*(6), 493-503. doi:10.5014/ajot.45.6.493

Florey, L. L. (1969). Intrinsic motivation: The dynamics of occupational therapy theory. *American Journal of Occupational Therapy, 23*(4), 319-322.

Grajo, L. (2017). Occupational adaptation. In J. Hinojosa, P. Kramer, & C. B. Royeen (Eds.), *Perspectives on human occupation: Theories underlying practice* (2nd ed., pp. 287-311). Philadelphia, PA: F.A. Davis.

Grajo, L., Boisselle, A., & DaLomba, E. (2018). Occupational adaptation as a construct: A scoping review of literature. *Open Journal of Occupational Therapy, 6*(1). doi:10.15453/2168-6408.1400

Grajo, L. & Cruz, D.M.C. (2017). Editorial: A hundred-year journey and a return to our roots—occupation, adaptation through occupation, and client-centeredness. *Cadernos Brasileiros de Terapia Ocupacional/Brazilian Journal of Occupational Therapy, 25*(3). doi: https://doi.org/10.4322/2526-8910.ctoED2503

Grajo, L. C., & Candler, C. (2016a). An occupation and participation approach to reading intervention (OPARI) part I: Defining reading as an occupation. *Journal of Occupational Therapy, Schools and Early Intervention, 9*(1), 74-85. doi:10.1080/19411243.2016.1141082

Grajo, L. C., & Candler, C. (2016b). An occupation and participation approach to reading intervention (OPARI) part II: Pilot clinical application. *Journal of Occupational Therapy, Schools and Early Intervention, 9*(1), 86-98. doi:10.1080/19411243.2016.1141083

Grajo, L., & Candler, C. (2017). The occupation and participation approach to reading intervention (OPARI): A community of practice study. *Journal of Occupational Therapy, Schools, and Early Intervention, 10*(1), 90-99. doi:10.1080/19411243.2016.1257967

Grajo, L., Candler, C., Lange, J., Cooseman, L., Sullivan, M., Breitenbucher, L., & Krumm, L. (2016). Well read: Community of practice helps occupational therapists support children with reading difficulties. *OT Practice, 21*(18), 8-14.

Kielhofner, G. (1977). Temporal adaptation: A conceptual framework for occupational therapy. *American Journal of Occupational Therapy, 31*(4), 235-242.

Kielhofner, G. (2009). *Conceptual foundations of occupational therapy practice* (4th ed.). Philadelphia, PA: F.A. Davis.

King, L. J. (1978). 1978 Eleanor Clarke Slagle Lecture: Toward a science of adaptive responses. *American Journal of Occupational Therapy, 32*(7), 429-437.

Kleinman, B. L., & Buckley, B. L. (1982). Some implications of a science of adaptive responses. *American Journal of Occupational Therapy, 36*, 16-19. doi:10.5014/ajot.36.1.15

Law, M., Baptiste, S., Cardswell, A., McColl, M. A., Polatajko, H., & Pollock, N. (2005). *Canadian occupational performance measure* (4th ed.). Ottawa, ON: CAOT Publications.

Llorens, L. A. (1970). Facilitating growth and development: The promise of occupational therapy. *American Journal of Occupational Therapy, 24*, 93-101.

Meyer, A. (1977). The philosophy of occupation therapy. *American Journal of Occupational Therapy, 31*(10), 639-642. (Reprinted from Archives of Occupational Therapy, 1922, 1, pp. 1-10.)

Nayar, S., & Stanley, M. (2014). Occupational adaptation as a social process in everyday life. *Journal of Occupational Science, 22*(1), 26-38. doi:10.1080/14427591.2014.882251

Nelson, D. L. (1988). Occupation: Form and performance. *American Journal of Occupational Therapy, 42*, 633-641. doi:10.5014/ajot.42.10.633

Reilly, M. (1962). Occupational therapy can be one of the greatest ideas of 20th century medicine (1961 Slagle Lecture). *American Journal of Occupational Therapy, 16*, 1-9.

Royeen, C., Grajo, L., & Luebben, A. (2014). Nonstandardized testing. In J. Hinojosa & P. Kramer (Eds.), *Evaluation in occupational therapy: Obtaining and interpreting data* (4th ed., pp. 121-141). Bethesda, MD: AOTA Press.

Schkade, J., & McClung, M. (2001). *Occupational adaptation in practice: Concepts and cases.* Thorofare, NJ: SLACK Incorporated.

Schkade, J. K., & Schultz, S. (1992). Occupational adaptation: Toward a holistic approach for contemporary practice, part 1. *American Journal of Occupational Therapy, 46*(9), 829-837. doi:10.5014/ajot.46.9.829

Schkade, J. K., & Schultz, S. (2003). Occupational adaptation. In P. Kramer, J. Hinojosa, & C. B. Royeen (Eds.), *Perspectives in human occupation: Participation in life* (pp. 181-221). Baltimore, MD: Lippincott Williams & Wilkins.

Schultz, S. (2014). Theory of occupational adaptation. In B. A. B. Schell, G. Gillen & M. E. Scaffa (Eds.), *Willard & Spackman's occupational therapy* (12th ed., pp. 527-540). Philadelphia, PA: Lippincott Williams & Wilkins.

Schultz, S., & Schkade, J. K. (1992). Occupational adaptation: Toward a holistic approach for contemporary practice, part 2. *American Journal of Occupational Therapy, 46*(10), 917-925. doi:10.5014/ajot.46.10.917

Schultz, S., & Schkade, J. K. (1997). Adaptation. In C. H. Christiansen & C. M. Baum (Eds.), *Occupational therapy: Enabling function and wellbeing* (2nd ed., pp. 458-481). Thorofare, NJ: SLACK Incorporated.

Soeker, M. S. (2011). Occupational adaptation: A return to work perspective of persons with mild to moderate brain injury in South Africa. *Journal of Occupational Science, 17*(1), 81-91. doi:10.1080/144275 91.2011.554155

Wenger, E. (2000). Communities of practice and social learning systems. *Organization, 7*(2), 225-246. doi:10.1177/135050840072002

White, R. W. (1959). Motivation reconsidered: The concept of competence. *Psychological Review, 66*, 297-333.

World Health Organization. (2001). *International Classification of Functioning, Disability and Health (ICF).* Geneva, Switzerland: Author.

Yerxa, E. J. (1967). Authentic occupational therapy (1966 Slagle Lecture). *American Journal of Occupational Therapy, 21*, 1-9.

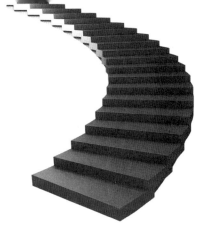

6

Formation of Identity and Occupational Competence
Occupational Adaptation in the Model of Human Occupation

Patricia Bowyer, EdD, MS, OTR, FAOTA

OVERVIEW This chapter defines occupational adaptation from the perspective of the Model of Human Occupation (MOHO). Occupational adaptation is a product of occupational identity, occupational competence, and the impact of the environment during occupational participation. MOHO organizes client factors to understand how a person approaches occupations. MOHO organizes occupational engagement through hierarchical and interrelated *dimensions of doing*, which include occupational participation, occupational performance, and occupational skills. As a person participates in daily occupations, the process of occupational adaptation occurs.

Grajo LC, Boisselle AK, eds.
Adaptation Through Occupation:
Multidimensional Perspectives (pp 105-121).
© 2019 SLACK Incorporated.

CHAPTER OBJECTIVES By the end of this chapter, the reader will be able to:

- Describe the constructs of MOHO.
- Describe the different dimensions of doing organized in MOHO.
- Define occupational adaptation, occupational identity, and occupational competence.
- Describe how change is viewed in MOHO and its effect on occupational adaptation, occupational identity, and occupational competence.
- Describe the empirical evidence and clinical application (assessments) of MOHO as linked to occupational identity and occupational competence on occupational adaptation.

QUESTIONS FOR DISCUSSION AND REFLECTION As the reader explores this chapter, let the following questions guide discussion and reflection:

- How can I use the language of occupational adaptation, competence, and identity in daily practice?
- How can I use MOHO in daily practice and articulate the impact of occupational therapy services in my client's process of adaptation?

INTRODUCTION

Occupation and adaptation are two tenets that ground occupational therapy practice. Within the field of occupational therapy, many theories and models have been developed to examine, explore, and explain occupation and adaptation. This chapter will discuss occupational adaptation as described in the MOHO (Taylor, 2017). Within MOHO, occupation and adaptation are central to the therapeutic relationship and occupational therapy process engaged in to impact the lives of individuals receiving the services of an occupational therapy practitioner. Although MOHO is organized around the concepts of *volition, habituation, performance capacity,* and the *influence of the environment* upon each, change in the therapeutic process occurs when an individual's occupational identity and/or occupational competence are impacted and the process of occupational adaptation occurs. MOHO provides a framework to organize the thinking and therapeutic approach undertaken by occupational therapy practitioners to address the occupational needs of clients being served. In order to engage with clients, occupational therapists using MOHO must (1) become familiar with the conceptual foundations of the model; (2) understand how these impact what MOHO describes as *dimensions of doing* (occupational participation, occupational performance, and occupational skills), which organizes human occupation; and (3) understand how change occurs within the person and the implications of change as it relates to occupational identity, occupational competence, and occupational adaptation (Taylor, 2017).

UNDERSTANDING THE CONCEPTUAL BEGINNINGS OF THE MODEL OF HUMAN OCCUPATION

MOHO evolved from the tradition of Reilly's occupational behavior theory (Kielhofner, 1980a, 1980b; Kielhofner & Burke, 1980; Kielhofner, Burke, & Igi, 1980). Dr. Gary Kielhofner trained with Dr. Mary Reilly as a graduate student at the University of Southern California (USC), which is when he began to develop his ideas about occupation and humans engaged in occupation. Dr. Kielhofner graduated from USC in 1974 with a master's degree in occupational therapy and then graduated from the University of California Los Angeles (UCLA) in 1980 with a doctorate of public health (Andersen & Reed, 2017). At this point in time, Kielhofner, Burke, and Igi published a series of four seminal articles outlining "the structure and content of a 'model of occupation'" (1980, p. 572). In the first article in the series, Kielhofner and Burke noted that occupational therapy was in a period of "crisis" because the profession did not have a "universal conceptual foundation to shape its identity and guide its practice"; rather, they noted, there was "a competition among proponents of alternative frames of reference for dominance in occupational therapy" and this had become "a crisis period in the development of the field" (1980, p. 572). Kielhofner and Burke (1980) expressed a desire for the "model of occupation" to be the "first step in the development of a paradigm for the field of occupational therapy" (p. 572). The aim was to present the MOHO as the unifying paradigm for the field and to provide a framework to be used in practice and research. In the initial publications outlining the MOHO, there are references to occupation (organized by subsystems), adaptation, change, competence, and identity (Kielhofner, 1980a, 1980b; Kielhofner & Burke, 1980; Kielhofner et al., 1980). MOHO was developed based on general systems theory; the constructs outlined in the 1980 model (Kielhofner, 1980a, 1980b, 1995, 2002, 2008; Kielhofner & Burke, 1980; Kielhofner et al., 1980) remain in the conceptual framework for the contemporary MOHO (Taylor, 2017). Although there has been refinement of the constructs, based on empirical investigation and application in clinical practice, the original constructs outlined remain, *volition, habituation, performance capacity,* and the *impact of the environment.* During the 38 years since the original publications on MOHO, numerous models of occupation have been developed for occupational therapy practitioners to use; however, to date, MOHO has the largest amount of empirical data to support its validity as a practice model and more assessments developed for use in practice than any other occupation model. Furthermore, occupational therapy practitioners have identified MOHO as the most frequently used model (Kielhofner, 2009; Lee, 2010; National Board for Certification in Occupational Therapy, 2004). This chapter is organized around the constructs of MOHO, the role of *doing* in organizing human occupation, and the way occupation and adaptation are viewed and linked to occupational identity and competence, with an overview of recent studies related to occupational identity, occupational competence, and occupational adaptation. It also presents assessments developed to identify concerns in these areas of a person's life.

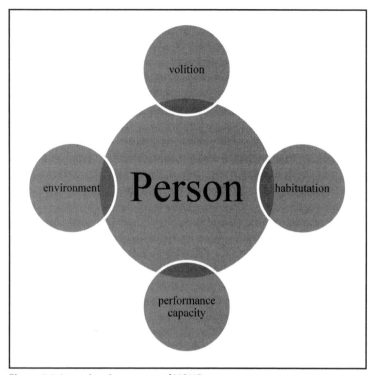

Figure 6-1. Interrelated constructs of MOHO.

MODEL OF HUMAN OCCUPATION CONSTRUCTS

MOHO comprises three interrelated constructs, which are organized to explain human behavior and the impact of the environment on it: volition, habituation, and performance *capacity*. These components lead to humans engaging in occupations (Figure 6-1).

Volition

Humans are driven to act; this drive to act is *volition* (Taylor, 2017). An individual's ability to act and engage in life, or occupation, is influenced by the underlying constructs of volition: *personal causation, values*, and *interests*. Personal causation is an individual's view of his ability to undertake an action and his or her perceived effectiveness of the action taken. When one engages in an occupation, one typically does so because of a belief that one is capable of performing it and that one will do so in an effective way. For example, an adult person has a desire to plant a container garden; although this person has planted gardens in the past, this is his first time planting a container garden. In reflecting on past experiences with planting a garden, he recalls success with effort. Therefore, he decides to act based on knowledge of a capacity, or capability, to undertake gardening in a new way because of being effective with gardening in the past. In this way, his thoughts and views on his ability to act lead him to engage in a desired life activity.

Another component of volition is the *value* placed on a given occupation or activity. Let's consider the impact of values on the adult person planting a container garden. Growing up in a rural environment, he planted a garden each spring with his family. The family placed great value on the garden because it provided sustenance for the family and was a time when they worked together toward a common goal. This led to him continuing the tradition of planting a garden with his own family. His family is now grown and moved out; he has no need to plant a large garden, but he still finds meaning and value in being able to grow vegetables, share them with others, and use them in the meals he prepares. At this point in his life, he no longer needs to plant a large garden because his children have grown and moved out.

A final component of volition is *interest*. In our example, the adult person was driven to act based on a positive sense of personal causation and a desire to engage in a valued occupation. Another factor in choosing to engage in an occupation is level of interest. Our adult person finds the idea of engaging in the occupation of a container garden to be satisfying and enjoyable. Because of these views of the occupation of a container garden, he has a desire to act. He derives pleasure in the act of obtaining the materials to create a container garden: pots, soil, seeds. Once he has completed this, he then derives joy in caring for the container garden: watering and fertilizing it. Finally, he has contentment at being able to share the vegetables he harvests with his neighbors and family. This results in him having an *interest* in engaging in the occupation of maintaining a container garden. These three subconstructs form volition, and it is through these components that action is taken to engage in occupation.

Habituation

Habituation is the "semi-autonomous patterning of behavior in concert with our familiar temporal, physical, and social habitats" (Taylor, 2017). The two components that comprise habituation are *habits* and *internalized roles*. Habits are patterns of behavior that are undertaken on an hourly, daily, weekly, monthly, and yearly basis. Within the temporal framework, habits become automatic actions based on time, place, and social group. For example, there is the pattern of a work or school day vs the pattern of a weekend day. During a work or school day, the pattern of behavior may include arising early in the morning and not returning home until late in the evening. During the day, there are various patterned occupations that are undertaken. A student attends class, has a lunch break, and then may participate in an after-school occupation. Within a given occupation, there are patterns of behavior. In the morning, one person may brush his teeth before taking a shower, whereas another brushes her teeth after taking a shower. Within the occupation of brushing teeth, there are the habits of how toothpaste is put on the brush (from front to back or from back to front), the temperature of the water used to brush the teeth (hot, warm, cold), and the way the brush is used (circular motion or up-and-down motion) to clean the teeth. With each of these patterns of behavior (habit) in occupation, there is an autopilot, an unconscious engagement because the occupation has been repeated hundreds of times in a lifetime.

Internalized roles are the other component of habituation. *Roles* are patterns of action that relate to a particular social status or identity (Taylor, 2017). A role is based upon the socialization for action or behavior that occurs by virtue of being in a particular social status. Roles are defined by internalized expectations and/or external expectations. For example, there are certain expectations that a stay-at-home mom has vs those of a working mother; the stay-at-home mom provides primary care for her children during an entire day, and hence this becomes her primary role identification. A working mom has dual role identities: that of a mom and a worker outside the home. Within each of these roles, there are different demands and expectations. Both mothers internalize and assume role identity based on the social expectations placed on being a mom, and a certain pattern of actions occur because of the role. For the working mom, there is also the identification of expectations for that role and the socialization that creates an internalized sense of expectations for the role and how it is defined. These two subconstructs form habituation and allow for the patterning of occupation throughout a person's day-to-day, week-to-week, month-to-month, and year-to-year life.

Performance Capacity and Environmental Impact

Performance capacity consists of the objective physical and mental components as understood by the subjective (lived body) experience (Kielhofner, 2008; Taylor, 2017). MOHO does not specifically address issues of performance capacity as do other models (e.g., biomechanical approach, sensory integration). If there are specific physical limitations, they are taken in to consideration with MOHO, but MOHO does not specifically address objective physical and mental components. *Performance capacity* is the "ability for doing things" given the underlying objective physical and mental components (Taylor, 2017, p. 19). An interpretation of the experience is engaged in through what is termed a "lived body." This is the experience of "being and knowing the world though a particular body" (Taylor, 2017, p. 77). Performance capacity occurs within an environment and is impacted by it. The environment includes the physical and social components and can be supportive, facilitating performance, or it can be filled with barriers, hindering performance. Therefore, the environmental impact either allows for or interferes with a person's ability to engage in occupation.

When a person engages in occupation, the outside view is the objective perspective and the view from the person being inside his or her own body is the subjective perspective. An example of this is a child with sensory processing difficulties. The child enjoys going to the park with his family and likes watching his siblings go down the slide. However, he does not want to go down the slide. When his parents ask him why he does not want to go down the slide, he states that he is afraid he will not stop at the bottom and will keep going down in to the earth. While, by all appearances, the child should be able to engage in the occupation of sliding, his lived body (subjective experience) is a limiting factor in his performance capacity. Or, if a child has severe cerebral palsy and is unable to maneuver his physical body, he may be unable to engage in a desired occupation as a result of a physical limitation (objective perspective). In each of these situations, the experience in a person's body, and possibly the environment, can impact performance capacity. *Performance capacity* is made up of the objective physical and mental components that make up a person and are impacted by the subjective experience and the environment.

Summary of Model of Human Occupation Constructs

MOHO provides a conceptual framework to understand occupation by focusing on person-centered constructs of volition, habituation, and performance capacity as impacted by the environment. Through this lens, MOHO considers a person's abilities or disabilities. MOHO provides a methodical, structured approach to consider the needs, wants, and desires of a person. MOHO is not a standalone model; rather, it is designed to be used as a complement to other models and theories (e.g., biomechanical, cognition). The conceptual components of MOHO guide occupational therapy practitioners in their thinking and understanding of a person and his or her desire for action, pattern of occupation, and ability to perform. Using the conceptual components of MOHO to understand a person and how person factors impact engagement in occupation, it is then necessary to organize, frame, and understand levels of doing.

ORGANIZING ACTIONS: MODEL OF HUMAN OCCUPATION AND DIMENSIONS OF DOING

Doing is occupation. Occupation is how a person engages in life. As discussed earlier in this chapter, a person is driven to action, or doing, based on his or her volition, habituation, and performance capacity and whether the environment facilitates (or not) engagement in occupation. MOHO organizes *doing* into three levels: occupational participation, occupational performance, and occupational skills (Taylor, 2017). The three levels can be viewed as hierarchical but ultimately are interrelated (Figure 6-2). The ability to engage in occupation is structured so that occupational participation has an expansive view of doing. *Occupational participation* is defined by wide categories of work, play/leisure, and the occupations that are part of engaging in one's life. *Occupational participation* occurs within context and is impacted by whether there are supports or barriers to participation in occupations. The supports or barriers can be physical, emotional, psychological, social, or relational in nature. In order for a person to be able to experience occupational participation, he or she requires occupational performance.

Occupational performance is the ability of a person to undertake discrete actions or steps in order to fulfill what is needed to participate in a chosen occupation. MOHO views occupational performance as engaging in occupational form (Kielhofner, 2008; Taylor, 2017). *Occupational form* is the discrete action that is necessary to engage in an occupation; it involves the steps required to experience occupational performance (Kielhofner, 2008; Taylor, 2017). For example, a person wants to take a trip. There are several discrete acts, or steps, that have to be undertaken in order for the trip to occur: decide where to go, purchase a ticket for the planned dates of travel, decide where to stay while away, reserve housing, and plan what to do while on the trip. Each of these different actions is an occupational form that makes up the entire act of going on a trip. A factor in occupational performance is occupational skill.

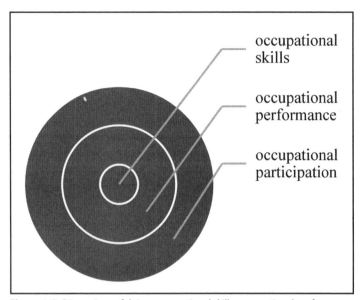

Figure 6-2. Dimensions of doing: occupational skills, occupational performance, and occupational participation.

Occupational skills are the "observable, goal-directed actions that make up occupational performance" (Taylor, 2017, p. 108). MOHO recognizes three types of skills: motor, process, and communication and interaction. *Motor skills* are the ability of a person to move his or her body or to engage in occupation and move objects in the environment. *Process skills* are a person's ability to decide on an activity to undertake, to organize the activity with the appropriate steps occurring as it is undertaken, to know what materials are needed, and to be able to use them appropriately to engage in the activity. *Communication and interaction skills* are a person's ability to express him- or herself in order to understand and be understood (Kielhofner, 2008; Taylor, 2017). Through occupational skills, a person is able to perform the discrete actions and steps needed to engage in an occupation, and in this way, he or she is able to achieve occupational performance and occupational participation. This ability to participate is done with the understanding that a person's volition, habituation, and performance capacity have a direct influence on what a person does, how he or she does it, when he or she does it, and why he or she does it. However, any of these levels of doing can be affected if a person experiences a debilitating injury or disease process. If this occurs, the person will need to go through the process of occupational adaptation. If a bakery owner has a hand injury that results in an inability to perform the motor skills necessary to make bread to sell in his shop, he may still be able to engage with his work through process skills and communication interaction skills by having the part-time worker in his store write out the list of materials needed for bread making and verbally sequencing the steps needed to mix the ingredients prior to baking the bread. Then, the part-time worker is able to provide the motor skills necessary to mix the ingredients and bake the bread. In this way, the baker is able to adapt to his current physical state in order to continue a valued role; thus, he is still able to attain all three levels of doing. However, if this were not the case, and a person was unable to overcome issues related to occupational skills, occupational performance, or occupational participation, there would be a need to identify the cause of the problem and then possibly seek assistance with occupational adaptation.

CHANGE: MODEL OF HUMAN OCCUPATION AND OCCUPATIONAL ADAPTATION AS MANIFESTED THROUGH OCCUPATIONAL IDENTITY AND OCCUPATIONAL COMPETENCE

Occupational adaptation has been a cornerstone to the field, even before occupational therapy became a formal professional discipline. Hall (1905) discussed the value of work-cure for individuals experiencing debilitating issues. In his practice, he observed the value of occupation of the mind and hands and the importance of adapting the occupation undertaken to meet the current state of his patients in order to move them forward toward a more engaged life. Tracy (1907) added to this view of adaptation, discussing the role of an engineer to adapt a weaving frame to allow a child to weave and make doll rugs and other woven items. She discussed the value of occupation and adaptation and the impact on the lives of her patients. A move forward in the history of the profession and occupational adaptation was described as the importance of man to engage in activity to improve his body and mind (Fidler & Fidler, 1978; Reilly, 1962). From these beginnings arose the foundations for the view of occupational adaptation within MOHO.

MOHO defines occupational adaptation as the achievement of an occupational identity and a sense of occupational competence as achieved over the span of time as influenced by the environment (Kielhofner, 2008; Taylor, 2017). The relationship, positive or negative, between occupational identity, occupational competence, and the environment is what results in occupational adaptation. It is through participation that a person is able to achieve a sense of occupational identity and occupational competence. This engagement can either be supported or hindered by the environment in which it occurs.

Occupational Identity

According to Christiansen (1999), an occupational identity is necessary to develop a person's self-awareness of desires, roles, relationships, values, and interests. By choosing to participate in various occupations, a person is able to form an occupational identity; in this way, the person gains an understanding of who he or she is, what he or she wants to achieve, and where he or she wants to go in life. An occupational identity is formed through a process of trial and error by engaging in chosen occupations and assessing the outcome, and then deciding to engage in the occupation again or to move on to a different occupation. Through this process, a person is using his or her volition to explore and engage in a desired occupation; then, the person assesses the outcome of the occupation (performance capacity) while deciding if the occupation is truly valued and of interest (habituation). It is through this ongoing process that participation is achieved and an occupational identity formed. An occupational identity provides a personal sense of self: who I am, what I value, what I find interesting and desirable to do. It is through this understanding of self that a person is able to organize his or her life around occupations that are desirable and begin a process of occupational adaptation (Kielhofner, 2008; Taylor, 2017). For example, a person has a desire to become a photographer. There is an initial desire to try this new occupation, but, if not acted upon, it cannot become part of her occupational identity. If acted upon, she has to decide how to go about becoming proficient at taking photographs. She may consider: "Do I want to do it as a leisure activity, or do I want to pursue it and choose to become a professional photographer?" Whatever the choice, the occupational identity that is formed as a result would be quite different: An occupational identity of photographer as a leisure pursuit would be very different from that of photographer as a career. A person choosing to pursue photography as a leisure activity may be willing to invest less money in the tools required to take photos and decide that an occasional course on photography is satisfying and provides enough information and support to lead to success in the chosen hobby. However, if she chooses to pursue photography as a career, the importance placed on the photos taken would be much more because the photos have to provide financial support. Therefore, she may decide to invest in the best photography equipment available and to take a series of courses leading to specialization in photography. Although the outcome for each choice is to become a photographer, there is significant difference in the meaning behind the occupation for each choice. An occupational identity is based on a subjective view of the outcomes of occupations and occupational participation. If a person finds that a chosen occupation achieves a desired outcome, then he or she will continue in it. If the results of participating in a chosen occupation do not achieve desired results, then the person may decide that the occupation is not to be desired or pursued, and it does not become part of an occupational identity.

Occupational Competence

Occupational competence reflects the meaning (occupational identity) given to chosen occupations. *Occupational competence* is the action that is required to fulfill the expectations attached to a role. Once a person chooses to pursue an occupation, the person then has to have a sense that he or she will be able to succeed in the chosen occupation. Occupational competence is the manifestation of an occupational identity; it is an ability to carry out a desired and chosen occupation. It is the sense that the capacity to perform an occupation exists and that, if undertaken, the outcome will be positive and successful. In the example of a person choosing to pursue photography as a career, she has to have a sense that she will be able to meet the expectations of a worker role as linked to a photographer. She needs to be able to perform at her expected standards for the role, follow the routines that are necessary to succeed in the role, and continue in what is expected until the desired life goal is realized (Kielhofner, 2008; Taylor, 2017). Through this process of meeting expectations for a role, she can achieve occupational competence.

Environment

A person's ability to participate in occupations is impacted by the environment and cannot be overlooked when examining the components involved with occupational adaptation; regardless of a person's occupational identity and occupational competence, environmental factors (physical, social, cultural, political, and economic) can either facilitate or hinder the pursuit of desired occupations (Kielhofner, 2008; Taylor, 2017). Let's consider the impact the environment can have on the person seeking to pursue photography as a leisure pursuit. An environmental consideration could be if she comes from a culture that does not agree with people or things being photographed. However, she has moved away from her culture of origin and been exposed to photography through visits to photo exhibits at museums. It is through these visits that she became interested in pursuing photography as a leisure occupation, having observed the beauty and meaning that can be derived from nature photos. Although she has a desire to purse photography and the physical capacity to perform the occupation, she will have to come to terms with a deep-seated cultural norm from her social environment and family. As she negotiates a desire to pursue the occupation (occupational identity), knowing she has the ability to undertake the occupation (occupational competence), she still may need to come to terms with the cultural environment of her origins in order to purse photography as a leisure outlet. Thus, according to MOHO, the environment must be factored in to understanding occupational adaptation.

Occupational Adaptation

In MOHO, occupational adaptation is "having a positive occupational identity and the corresponding occupational competence, constructed over time through the dynamics of a constant interaction between personal factors and environmental impact" (Taylor, 2017, p. 118). As people develop throughout a lifetime, there can be phases of occupational adaptation. As a child, a person is learning how to do the things that are part of childhood: being a daughter to a parent, learning to dress and groom, and being a friend. Then, in early childhood into adolescence, this expands. During this phase of life, a person is learning how to be a student, possibly a worker, and to engage in pastime activities that are of interest. Then, moving into being an adult, additional life occupations are learned and undertaken: being a worker, parent, spouse, community member, and volunteer and continuing to engage in preferred leisure activities and possibly pursue additional new ones. Throughout a person's life, there is a constant interplay between volition, habituation, performance skills, and how the environment is affecting a person's ability to participate and his or her occupational identity and occupational competence. It is through these components that life unfolds and that occupational adaptation, as a process, occurs. The interaction of personal factors and the environment lead to participation in a chosen occupation, and, through this, occupational identity and occupational competence are established. The result of the interactions of all of these aspects combined is a state of occupational adaptation. Occupational adaptation occurs naturally as people pass through life phases. However, there are times when life circumstances result in a disability from an illness or accident, and this can lead to a disruption in a person's occupational identity and occupational competence. In each of these instances, it is important to understand the impact of change. Change, whether positive or as the result of something that could be deemed negative, is inevitable in life. Change factors into occupational adaptation and how people participate in occupations.

Change and Occupational Adaptation

Change naturally occurs as people move through life. There is an "ongoing process of change" as people develop (Taylor, 2017, p. 148). Kielhofner (2008) describes three different types of change that can occur in a person's lifetime: incremental, catastrophic, and transformational. *Incremental change* is the small change that occurs just because a person is alive. These are the day-in, day-out changes that are experienced. These can be seen in the young child beginning to crawl and then moving on to walking or in the older person who begins to feel the arthritic changes in his joints and moves more slowly when walking. Change can also be catastrophic. A *catastrophic change* is one that occurs unexpectedly and results in a major change in abilities or roles. This can happen when a person is laid off from a job and is no longer in a worker role or when a person has an accident that results in a physical disability. This affects the person's physical capabilities, but it can also impact roles and role expectations. Finally, *transformational change* occurs when a person makes a conscious decision to pursue a new occupation or add a new role, or when he or she decides a current role is no longer valued and discontinues it.

In each of these cases of change, occupational adaptation is occurring. Incremental change can be observed as a child grows. There is a desire to explore and master the environment, and this allows for a sense of occupational identity and occupational competence to emerge, leading to occupational adaptation, as noted by the child's participating in desired occupations. An adolescent seeking employment must find a job, fill out an application, participate in an interview, and accept a job if offered. Through these experiences, the adolescent is gaining a new occupational identity and confirming the same through occupational competence, resulting in occupational adaptation. Catastrophic change can be noted in the life of an adult who experiences an accident and is left with an inability to fulfill role obligations because of physical limitations. In this situation, the adult can either adjust (adapt) to the change in role and role expectations and move forward in life or become debilitated by the loss and be unable to adapt to the change. Finally, there is transformational change. A person experiencing transformational change has consciously acknowledged a need to make a change. This person is going to adjust his or her occupational identity and occupational competence to accept the change and move on to occupational adaptation.

Occupational adaptation is derived from the need for change in order to participate in one's own life. The need to enable occupational participation in life is centered on change, and change comes in various forms. Occupational adaptation can occur naturally (incremental), be the result of an unexpected occurrence (catastrophic), or be made consciously with an understanding of the possible implications for the decision and choice made (transformational). In all of these cases of change, occupational identity and occupational competence as influenced by volition, habituation, and performance capacity as impacted by the environment lead to occupational adaptation. However, at times there is the need to aid in understanding the change that has occurred or is occurring. More likely than not, a clinician will encounter a person who has experienced catastrophic change. In an effort to aid in understanding the personal and environmental factors impacted by this change and how it is affecting occupational participation and occupational adaptation, a number of assessments based on MOHO components as linked to these factors have been developed. Each provides a specific focus and can be an aid in guiding thinking about the occupational needs of clients served.

OPERATIONALIZE: MODEL OF HUMAN OCCUPATION TOOLS TO GUIDE PRACTICE

A number of assessments have been developed to measure the components of MOHO. For the purposes of this chapter, six of the assessments are included in Table 6-1. The assessments included provide measures of participation, various age groups, different MOHO domains, and styles of administration. The selection of a MOHO assessment should take each of these factors into consideration. However, it is recommended that in most cases, either the Model of Human Occupation Screening Tool (MOHOST) (Parkinson, Forsyth, & Kielhofner, 2006) or the Short Child Occupational Profile (SCOPE; Bowyer et al., 2008) be used first to establish a baseline and an occupational profile. An occupational profile provides details about a person's occupational interests, patterns of activity, routines, and occupational life history. Additionally, it is possible that once the MOHOST or SCOPE has been administered, it may be found to guide the clinician to use another MOHO assessment that focuses more closely on a specific component of MOHO. The MOHOST and the SCOPE are global assessments based on all of the components of MOHO and are designed to provide a holistic understanding of a client and a client's level of occupational participation. MOHO assessments are outlined by Taylor (2017) and are easily accessible on the Model of Human Occupation Clearinghouse website (www.cade.uic.edu/moho).

ADVANCING THE KNOWLEDGE ON OCCUPATIONAL ADAPTATION

Clinicians can use the evidence in Table 6-2 to understand how MOHO components have been examined empirically as linked to occupational adaptation, occupational identity, and occupational competence. The evidence provided is not exhaustive and represents more recent studies. For a more expansive review of the evidence on MOHO, access Model of Human Occupation Clearinghouse website (www.cade.uic.edu/moho) for research briefs. There is also a section in Taylor's Kielhofner's *Model of Human Occupation* (2017) that outlines the various domains and components of the model.

Table 6-1

Model of Human Occupation Assessments			
Assessment	**Age Range**	**Method**	**Purpose**
Model of Human Occupation Screening Tool (MOHOST) (Parkinson et al., 2006)	Adolescent to adult	Interview, observation, chart review, other assessments	The MOHOST is an assessment that addresses the majority of MOHO concepts with which a therapist can gain an overview of the client's occupational participation.
Short Child Occupational Profile (SCOPE) (Bowyer et al., 2008)	Child to adolescent	Interview, observation, chart review, other assessments	The SCOPE is an occupation-focused assessment that measures factors linked to occupational participation.
Child Occupational Self-Assessment (COSA) (Kramer et al., 2014)	Child to adolescent	Self-rated	The COSA is a client-directed assessment designed to capture perceptions regarding occupational competence and the importance of everyday activities.
Occupational Self-Assessment (OSA) (Baron, Kielhofner, Iyenger, Goldhammer, & Wolenski, 2006)	Adolescent to adult	Self-rated	The OSA is designed to capture clients' perceptions of their own occupational competence on their occupational adaptation.
Occupational Performance History Interview-II (OPHI-II) (Kielhofner et al., 2004)	Adolescent to adult	Semi-structured interview	The OPHI-II explores a client's life history in the areas of work, play, and self-care performance.
The Occupational Circumstances Assessment Interview and Rating Scale (OCAIRS) (Forsyth et al., 2005)	Adolescent to adult	Semi-structured interview	The OCAIRS gathers information on the extent and nature of an individual's occupational participation.

Table 6-2

Recent Model of Human Occupation Evidence Occupational Identity, Occupational Competence, and Occupational Adaptation		
Year Published	Authors	Summary
2013	Nygren, Sandlund, Bernspang, & Fisher	This study examined the perceptions of occupational competence and occupational value among individuals with mental illness in Sweden.
2013	Williams & Murray	An interpretive phenomenological approach was undertaken to examine the lived experience of occupational adaptation with clients following a stroke.
2013	Sandell, Kjellberg, & Taylor	This study examined the impact of a diagnosis of autism spectrum disorder or attention deficit hyperactivity disorder on a person's occupational identity and occupational competence and the interaction with the environment.
2012	Costa & Othero	The authors examined use of MOHO within the context of palliative care; the focus was on assisting clients to regain an occupational identity.
2011	Johansson & Isaksson	A qualitative study was undertaken to examine the impact of extended sick leave on occupational adaptation, occupational identity, and occupational competence.

SUMMARY AND IMPLICATIONS

- MOHO provides a framework to aid in understanding the clinical implications linked to occupational adaptation.
- The person factors as presented by MOHO (volition, habituation, and performance capacity) are involved in the development of occupational identity and occupational competence, leading to life participation and occupational adaptation.
- Participation and occupational adaptation are impacted by change, either positive or negative. Understanding the type of change that occurs (incremental, catastrophic, or transformational) can serve as a guide to attaining or meeting the occupational needs of clients.
- The assessments developed for use with MOHO allow clinicians to systematically examine the personal and environmental factors impacting occupational adaptation of their clients.
- Recent evidence has been generated to support the use of MOHO in clinical practice and specifically to address occupational adaptation as impacted by occupation identity and occupational competence.

REFERENCES

Andersen, L. T., & Reed, K. L. (2017). *The history of occupational therapy: The first century*. Thorofare, NJ: SLACK Incorporated.

Baron, K., Kielhofner, G., Iyenger, A., Goldhammer, V., & Wolenski, J. (2006). *Occupational Self-Assessment (OSA) (Version 2.2)* [Assessment]. Chicago, IL: University of Illinois at Chicago. Retrieved from https://www.moho.uic.edu/productDetails.aspx?aid=2

Bowyer, P. L., Kramer, J., Ploszaj, A., Ross, M., Schwartz, O., Kielhofner, G., & Kramer, K. (2008). *The Short Child Occupational Profile (SCOPE) (Version 2.2)* [Assessment]. Chicago, IL: University of Illinois at Chicago. Retrieved from https://www.moho.uic.edu/productDetails.aspx?aid=9

Christiansen, C. H. (1999). Defining lives: Occupation as identity: An essay on competence, coherence and the creation of meaning. *American Journal of Occupational Therapy, 53*(6), 547-558.

Costa, A., & Othero, M. (2012). Palliative care, terminal illness, and the model of human occupation. *Physical and Occupational Therapy in Geriatrics, 30*(4), 316-327.

Fidler, G. S., & Fidler, J. W. (1978). Doing and becoming: Purposeful action and self-actualization. *American Journal of Occupational Therapy, 32*, 305-310.

Forsyth, K., Deshpande, S., Kielhofner, G., Henriksson, C., Haglund, L., Olson, L., … Kulkarni, S. (2005). The Occupational Circumstances Assessment Interview and Rating Scale (OCAIRS) (Version 4.0) [Assessment]. Chicago, IL: University of Illinois at Chicago. Retrieved from https://www.moho.uic.edu/productDetails.aspx?aid=35

Hall, H. J. (1905). Neurasthenia. A study of etiology. Treatment by occupation. *Boston Medical and Surgical Journal, CLIII*(2), 47-49.

Johansson, C., & Isaksson, G. (2011). Experiences of participation in occupations of women on long-term sick leave. *Scandinavian Journal of Occupational Therapy, 18*, 294-301.

Kielhofner, G. (1980a). A model of human occupation, part 2. *American Journal of Occupational Therapy, 34*(10), 657-663.

Kielhofner, G. (1980b). A model of human occupation, part 3. *American Journal of Occupational Therapy, 34*(11), 731-737.

Kielhofner, G. (1995). *A model of human occupation: Theory and application* (2nd ed.). Baltimore, MD: Lippincott Williams & Wilkins.

Kielhofner, G. (2002). *A model of human occupation: Theory and application* (3rd ed.). Philadelphia, PA: Lippincott Williams & Wilkins.

Kielhofner, G. (2008). *A model of human occupation: Theory and application* (4th ed.). Philadelphia, PA: Lippincott Williams & Wilkins.

Kielhofner, G. (2009). *Conceptual foundations of occupational therapy practice* (4th ed.). Philadelphia, PA: F.A. Davis.

Kielhofner, G., & Burke, J. (1980). A model of human occupation, part 1. *American Journal of Occupational Therapy, 34*(9), 572-581.

Kielhofner, G., Burke, J., & Igi, C. (1980). A model of human occupation, part 4. *American Journal of Occupational Therapy, 34*(12), 777-788.

Kielhofner, G., Mallinson, T., Crawford, C., Nowak, M., Rigby, M., Henry, A., & Walens, D. (2004). *The Occupational Performance History Interview-II (OPHI-II) (Version 2.1)* [Assessment]. Chicago, IL: University of Illinois at Chicago. Retrieved from https://www.moho.uic.edu/productDetails.aspx?aid=31

Kramer, J., ten Velden, M., Kafkes, A., Basu, S., Federico, J., & Kielhofner, G. (2014). *Child Occupational Self-Assessment (COSA) (Version 2.2)* [Assessment]. Chicago, IL: University of Illinois at Chicago. Retrieved from https://www.moho.uic.edu/productDetails.aspx?aid=3

Lee, J. (2010). Achieving best practice: A review of evidence linked to occupation-focused practice models. *Occupational Therapy in Health Care, 24*(3), 206-222.

National Board for Certification in Occupational Therapy. (2004). A practice analysis study of entry-level occupational therapist registered and certified occupational therapy assistant practice. *OTJR: Occupation, Participation, and Health, 24*(Suppl. 1), S1-S31.

Nygren, U., Sandlund, M., Bernspang, B., & Fisher, A. (2013). Exploring the perceptions of occupational competence among participants in individual placement and support (IPS). *Scandinavian Journal of Occupational Therapy, 20,* 429-437.

Parkinson, S., Forsyth, K., & Kielhofner, G. (2006). *The Model of Human Occupation Screening Tool (MOHOST) (Version 2.0)* [Assessment]. Chicago, IL: University of Illinois at Chicago. Retrieved from https://www.moho.uic.edu/productDetails.aspx?aid=4

Reilly, M. (1962). Occupational therapy can be one of the great ideas of 20th century medicine. *American Journal of Occupational Therapy, 16,* 1-9.

Sandell, C., Kjellberg, A., & Taylor, R. (2013). Participating in diagnostic experience: Adults with neuro-psychiatric disorders. *Scandinavian Journal of Occupational Therapy, 20,* 136-142.

Taylor, R. (Ed.). (2017). *Kielhofner's model of human occupation* (5th ed.). Philadelphia, PA: Wolters Kluwer.

Tracy, S. E. (1907). Some profitable occupations for invalids. *American Journal of Nursing, 8,* 172-177.

Williams, S., & Murray, C. (2013). The lived experience of older adults' occupational adaptation following a stroke. *Australian Occupational Therapy Journal, 60,* 39-47.

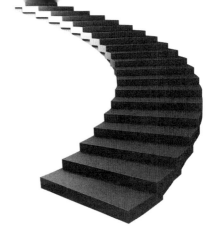

7

Adaptation From a Sensory Processing Perspective

Lauren Little, PhD, OTR/L and Winifred Dunn, PhD, OTR, FAOTA

OVERVIEW In this chapter, occupational adaptation is framed within a sensory processing perspective. Sensory processing is a fundamental feature of the human experience that informs us about our bodies and the world around us. Drawing from neuroscience literature, research shows that there is variability in how individuals sense and respond to sensory information in their environments. When persons receive different sensory input or interpret sensory input differently, those persons' behaviors will reflect those differences.

When persons respond based on the sensory experiences they are having, we might call this their adaptive response, although the behaviors may not be useful in context. We support persons' adaptation by informing them, their families and friends, and other providers the characteristics of their sensory patterns so they can explore how those patterns impact everyday life.

Grajo LC, Boisselle AK, eds.
Adaptation Through Occupation:
Multidimensional Perspectives (pp 123-140).
© 2019 SLACK Incorporated.

CHAPTER OBJECTIVES By the end of this chapter, the reader will be able to:

- Describe the current research as well as historical perspectives about sensory processing and its impact on everyday life.
- Describe how sensory processing is a person characteristic that results in adaptive responses.
- Link sensory processing to both adaptive responses and functional participation.
- Describe the neuroscience literature that supports sensory processing as a person's adaptive response.
- Design strategies for improving adaptation and participation by adjusting activities and environments to support sensory processing patterns.

QUESTIONS FOR DISCUSSION AND REFLECTION As the reader explores this chapter, let the following questions guide discussion and reflection:

- How can I describe to clients and families the process of adaptation from a sensory processing perspective?
- How can I articulate the evidence for and impact on occupational adaptation of sensory processing interventions?

INTRODUCTION

Occupational adaptation is the experiential process by which individuals develop skills necessary to perform within their everyday environment (Gilfoyle, Grady, & Moore, 1981). From this viewpoint, the environment is a primary stimulus for development throughout the life span, and overall elements of occupational adaptation include the person, the environment, and the interaction of the person-environment during an occupation. *Sensory processing* refers to the ways in which individual person factors (i.e., detection and response to sensory stimuli) interact with the sensory stimuli in the environment and the attributes of the task. Individuals have unique sensory preferences and aversions, and their behavioral responses to environmental sensory stimuli reflect how they are adapting. When we do not understand individuals' behaviors, or label such behaviors as ineffective or maladaptive, it may be a clear mismatch between the person and environment sensory factors.

In the context of occupational adaptation, sensory processing must be considered as process based and nonhierarchical (Schkade & Schultz, 1992). That is, individuals' sensory processing preferences and aversions must not be considered as disorder or dysfunction; instead, the process of adaptation allows for individuals to match environments and personal strategies to activities. For example, an individual can gain coping strategies to mitigate negative sensory experiences and subsequently participate in meaningful activities. At a loud concert, an individual may discover that the use of earplugs supports her participation in the occupation. In this way, discovering how one's sensory preferences and aversions can be supported through environmental adaptations is considered process based. Sensory processing cannot be conceptualized as a hierarchical skill because sensory preferences and strategies are highly individualized and not universally linked to better or worse outcomes. Although there is a developmental timeline of how senses mature, the process of occupational adaptation with regard to sensory processing does not follow a set path. Because occupational adaptation emphasizes the individual's unique experience in the context of occupation, we must consider how one's sensory preferences and aversions both support and inhibit a person's choice of activities. Meaningful occupations are central to occupational adaptation. When individuals' sensory processing preferences and aversions do not match task demands, their participation is impacted.

The purpose of this chapter is to provide an overview of sensory processing as it relates to occupational adaptation. Although we acknowledge that cognitive and motor skills are linked to sensory processing, it is beyond the realm of this chapter to discuss cognitive and motor development; therefore, we will solely focus on adaptation from a sensory processing point of view. First, we discuss historical perspectives and contemporary models of sensory processing. Second, we provide an overview of current evidence related to sensory processing and cover the research on how sensory processing is linked to adaptive behaviors and participation across different populations. Third, we present findings from the neuroscience literature, which has investigated the underlying mechanisms of sensory processing. Finally, we discuss the evidence related to interventions that use sensory processing knowledge to promote participation, with an emphasis on how therapists can use strategies in natural contexts to support individuals' sensory processing patterns.

TERMINOLOGY

There are various terms that describe sensory processing, and terminology can become confusing because researchers from different disciplines use different terms. Because there is growing interest in sensory processing, some researchers have attempted to clarify differing terminology and assessment approaches, particularly between neuroscientists and occupational therapists (Baranek, Little, Parham, Ausderau, & Sabatos-DeVito, 2014; Cascio, Woynaroski, Baranek, & Wallace, 2016; Schaaf & Lane, 2015). Although we will use terms that describe specific sensory responses (e.g., *sensitivities, avoiding, seeking, registration*), we use the terms *sensory processing differences* and *sensory features* to capture the range of sensory experiences among individuals with and without conditions. We will discuss literature related to sensory processing differences among those with conditions (e.g., attention deficit hyperactivity disorder [ADHD], autism spectrum disorder [ASD]); however, such differences are not to be considered as deficits, abnormalities, or dysfunction. In fact, recent evidence suggests that people's sensory processing differences may be strengths and support participation in some activities (Bouvet, Mottron, Valdois, & Donnadieu, 2016; Little, Ausderau, Sideris, & Baranek, 2015).

Historical Perspectives of Sensory Processing

In 1972, Jean Ayres, an occupational therapist, defined sensory integration as "the organization of sensory information for use" (p. 1). Ayres described a theory of sensory integration in which children who had difficulty integrating sensory information also showed difficulty with purposeful behaviors such as learning new skills, regulating attention, and participating in school and home activities. Ayres was innovative because she used knowledge from neuroscience to help occupational therapists try to understand how children's behaviors may be related to their brains' ability to process sensory information and then produce an adaptive response. Ayres (1976) created the Southern California Sensory Integration Tests (SCSIT), evidence from which led early ideas of the application of sensory integration in children's lives. Based on evolving ideas, she then created the Sensory Integration and Praxis Tests (SIPT; Ayres, 1989), which includes 17 subtests designed to detect differences in sensory processes (e.g., visual perception, tactile perception, vestibular-proprioceptive functions) in children 4 to 9 years old. Although the SIPT aided practitioners and researchers when it was created, it is quite lengthy and costly and requires extensive training; therefore, the SIPT is not currently used widely in practice.

While sensory integration theory was gaining traction, Lorna Jean King was working with individuals with mental health conditions such as schizophrenia. King became interested in using principles from sensory integration theory to guide intervention with clients with mental health conditions as well as other conditions in children (e.g., dyslexia, ASD) (King, 1974, 1987). From Ayres' and King's research, the discipline of occupational therapy established the groundwork for understanding how sensory processing impacted participation among a variety of populations.

Contemporary Models of Sensory Processing

In 1997, Dunn proposed a Model of Sensory Processing describing the interaction of individual sensory detection thresholds (i.e., how quickly one detects) and self-regulation strategies (i.e., one's behavioral responses). Since then, Dunn has updated her Model of Sensory Processing. In Dunn's Sensory Processing Framework (Figure 7-1; Dunn, 2014), thresholds range from high (slow to detect) to low (quick to detect), and self-regulation ranges from passive to active. These two continua interact to create four sensory processing patterns: registration (high threshold and passive self-regulation), seeking (high threshold and active self-regulation), sensitivity (low threshold and passive self-regulation), and avoiding (low threshold and active self-regulation). Registration, also referred to as *hyporesponsiveness*, is characterized by a delayed or diminished detection of sensory

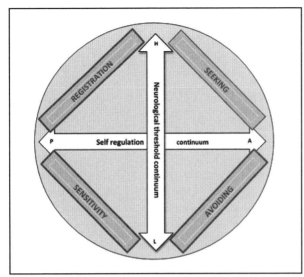

Figure 7-1. Dunn's Sensory Processing Framework. (Sensory Profile™ 2. Copyright © 2014 NCS Pearson, Inc. Reproduced with permission. All rights reserved. "Sensory Profile" is a trademark, in the US and/or other countries, of Pearson Education, Inc. or its affiliate[s].)

stimuli. Sensory-seeking behaviors include active involvement in activities or actions that provide intense sensory input. Avoidance/sensitivity, sometimes referred to as *hyper-responsiveness*, is characterized by an aversion to sensory stimuli. Although differences in sensory processing occur across systems (e.g., tactile and auditory), sensory processing patterns reflect behaviors that often occur across modalities and reflect thresholds and self-regulation strategies (Dunn, 2014).

There is differing terminology to describe sensory features across studies and fields, including *sensory under- and over-responsivity, hypo- and hyper-responsiveness, hypo- and hyper-reactivity,* and *sensory defensiveness* (Baranek et al., 2014; Schaaf & Lane, 2015). Overall, we use the terms as defined by Dunn's Sensory Processing Framework, which reflects sensory processing patterns, or those clusters of behaviors representative of detection thresholds (i.e., how quickly one detects) and self-regulation strategies (i.e., one's behavioral responses). Dunn, Little, Dean, Robertson, and Evans (2016) completed a scoping review to provide an overview of the evidence related to sensory processing and participation among children, and the findings suggest that the most highly used model is Dunn's Sensory Processing Framework; thus, we feel assured that the discussion here reflects current research.

STRUCTURES FOR ORGANIZING SENSORY PROCESSING KNOWLEDGE

There is great heterogeneity in sensory features both across diagnostic groups and in typical development (Baranek et al., 2014). Evidence suggests that sensory processing patterns differentially co-occur within and across individuals; they show sensitivities, avoiding, seeking, and registration patterns based on activity demands and contexts (Baranek et al., 2014; Little et al., 2015). Individuals' behavior is affected by the environment, and when individuals are in different situations, they likely show varying sensory preferences and aversions. For example, an empty train car is not likely to expose a person's aversion to touch from bumping into other people; a crowded train car would activate reactions to all the bumping.

When an individual shows different sensory responses in different environments, he or she may have to use a variety of strategies to increase adaptation across those environments. One study using the Sensory Profile (Dunn, 1999) showed that parents and teachers rated children differently (Brown & Dunn, 2010). This suggests that children may show differences in their sensory-related behaviors based on contextual characteristics. For example, children may be more hyper-responsive at school or engage in more sensory seeking due to the noise in the environment and the number of other children. First-hand accounts from those with ASD (Grandin & Scariano, 1986) suggest that busy, multisensory, and social environments may become overstimulating. Such overstimulation results in some individuals becoming withdrawn or unable to pick out the most relevant sensory stimuli.

Because there is increased evidence about the heterogeneity of sensory processing, researchers have created various structures for organizing sensory processing knowledge. That is, studies have tried to uncover how specific sensory processing patterns may help distinguish groups or characterize groups of people. Researchers have attempted to understand how sensory features may cluster together to characterize different types of people based on their sensory responses. For example, Miller, Anzalone, Lane, Cermak, and Osten (2007) proposed a nosology of sensory processing characteristics in an attempt to characterize children as having sensory modulation disorder, sensory-based motor disorder, sensory discrimination disorder.

Later, researchers focused on how sensory subtypes, or groupings of children, may characterize children with a diagnosis of ASD. Lane, Molloy, and Bishop (2014) used the Short Sensory Profile to uncover sensory subtypes of children with ASD. This study found four subtypes: (1) sensory adaptive, (2) taste-smell sensitive, (3) postural inattentive, and (4) generalized sensory difference. Ausderau et al. (2014) used the Sensory Experiences Questionnaire 3.0 (Baranek, 2009) to characterize sensory subtypes in a large sample of children with ASD. The researchers also found four subtypes: (1) mild, (2) sensitive-distressed, (3) attenuated-preoccupied, and (4) extreme-mixed. Although different parent questionnaires were used, both studies found that four subtypes best captured the variability in sensory processing patterns of children with ASD. Subtypes were characterized by the overall intensity of sensory features (e.g., sensory adaptive and mild, generalized sensory difference, and extreme-mixed) as well as the different co-occurrence of sensory processing patterns and modalities (e.g., taste-smell sensitive, postural inattentive, sensitive-distressed, attenuated-preoccupied). Specifically, the mild group was similar to the sensory adaptive group; these children with ASD showed very few sensory processing differences. The second group of children, sensitive-distressed, were somewhat similar to the taste-smell sensitive. Children in this group showed high rates of sensory sensitivities, particularly in taste and olfactory processing. Another group of children, attenuated-preoccupied, were similar to the postural inattentive group. This group showed high rates of sensory seeking and registration. Finally, the extreme-mixed group was similar to the generalized sensory difference group. Children in this group showed high rates of sensory processing differences across all sensory processing patterns.

Although research about sensory subtypes in ASD provides valuable information about that population, sensory processing patterns occur across the general population, including those with and without conditions (Dunn, Dean, Little, & Tomchek, 2018). Therefore, Little et al. (2015) investigated how the Sensory Profile-2 may characterize children in the general population. The researchers found five subtypes: (1) balanced, (2) interested, (3) intense, (4) mellow until..., and (5) vigilant. These subtypes varied by the intensity of sensory responses and the distribution of sensory features across the subtypes. The balanced sensory profile showed overall low sensory processing scores, whereas the intense sensory profile showed high sensory scores. The vigilant sensory profile showed increased sensitivity and avoidance to sensory stimuli, with low seeking and registration scores. The mellow until... sensory profile showed a high frequency of registration (i.e., misses more sensory cues) and avoidance, whereas the interested sensory profile was characterized by high rates of sensory seeking, with low scores on other sensory patterns. All five subtypes included children with and without conditions, such as ASD, ADHD, learning disabilities, and typical development. The findings suggest that sensory subtypes reflect the variability in all children, not just those with conditions. Future research may continue to investigate how the variability in sensory responses across individuals in the general population, as well as those with ASD, may be used to characterize groups.

CURRENT EVIDENCE OF SENSORY PROCESSING AND ADAPTATION

This section will provide an overview of evidence related to sensory processing differences among children with conditions and summarize findings from studies about how sensory processing is linked to adaptive behaviors and participation across different populations.

Extensive literature suggests that children with conditions differ from those without conditions on measures of sensory processing. Dunn et al. (2016) completed a scoping review to provide an overview of the evidence related to sensory processing and participation among children. The authors found that approximately 20% of research conducted on this topic between 2005 and 2015 was focused on the differences between populations of children based on measures of sensory processing. For example, many studies have compared sensory processing characteristics of those with ASD, typical development, and other developmental conditions. Studies suggest that as compared with typical development, children with ASD show increased rates of registration difficulties (Ben-Sasson et al., 2007; Watson et al., 2011) and hyper-responsiveness (Baranek, Boyd, Poe, David, & Watson, 2007). Some studies, however, suggest that the sensory processing characteristics of children with ASD do not differ from those with ADHD (Cheung & Siu, 2009). Children with fetal alcohol spectrum disorder have also been found to show differences in overall sensory processing (Jirikowic, Olson, & Kartin, 2008).

Other research has focused on how children with ADHD differ from those with typical development on sensory processing scores. Dunn and Bennett (2002), using the Sensory Profile (Dunn, 1999), found that children with ADHD differed from typically developing peers on sensory seeking, emotional reactivity, and inattention-distractibility. In partial support of these findings, Yochman, Parush, and Ornoy (2004) found that preschool-aged children with ADHD differed from those with typical development on seeking and oral sensitivity as well as auditory and visual processing; however, the ADHD group was not found to significantly differ on registration. Additionally, Pfeiffer, Daly, Nicholls, and Gullo (2015), using the Sensory Processing Measure (Parham & Ecker, 2007), found that children with ADHD demonstrated increased sensory processing scores as compared with those without ADHD.

Given these sensory processing differences among children with conditions, researchers have linked such sensory processing differences with activity participation and adaptive behavior. Activities provide structure for children and provide opportunities to understand themselves and their contexts as they learn and grow (Dunst et al., 2001; Humphry & Wakeford, 2008). Not surprisingly, children with ASD have lower frequency and variety of participation when compared with other children (Hilton, Graver, & LaVesser, 2007; Orsmond & Kuo, 2011). When children with ASD have high levels of hyper-responsiveness, they participate less frequently in social and community activities (Little et al., 2015). Carter, Ben-Sasson, and Briggs-Gowan (2011) also found that children's hyper-responsiveness was related to decreased activity particpation among families of children without conditions. Researchers have also reported that families participate in activities differently related to the children's sensory processing patterns. Studies have found that parents of children with ASD chose certain activities based on their children's sensory preferences and aversions (Bagby, Dickie, & Baranek, 2012; Schaaf, Toth-Cohen, Johnson, Outten, & Benevides, 2011). Additionally, participation is easier with family and a few close friends when children have differences in sensory processing (Cosbey, Johnston, & Dunn, 2010). Hochhauser and Engel-Yeger (2010) found that increased sensory features were associated with lower participation in social and physical activities. Although sensory characteristics have been associated with decreased participation in some studies, Little et al. (2015) found that enhanced perception (i.e., heighted sensory acuity) was associated with higher rates of participation in many activities for children with ASD.

Areas of occupation such as eating, sleep, and self-care are impacted when children have differences in sensory processing patterns. For example, children with ASD are often highly picky eaters and light sleepers; their patterns of hyper-responsive sensory processing are hypothesized as contributing factors (Nadon, Feldman, Dunn, & Gisel, 2011). Additionally, difficulties with communication and socialization in ASD have been associated with sensory hypo-responsiveness and sensory-seeking patterns (Baker, Lane, Angley, & Young, 2008; Jasmin et al., 2009; Liss, Saulnier, Fein, & Kinsbourne, 2006; Reynolds, Bendixen, Lawrence, & Lane, 2011). In typical development, avoidance is related to anxiety (Farrow & Coulthard, 2012) and sleep difficulties (Shochat, Tzischinsky, & Engel-Yeger, 2009).

Neurobiological Supports for Sensory Processing Knowledge

Increasing evidence suggests that individuals' sensory processing reflects a transactional relationship between individuals' biological traits and their context. Additionally, research suggests a developmental course to the integration of sensory information, which likely facilitates occupational adaptation. In this section, we present findings from the literature that has investigated the underlying biological and neural mechanisms of sensory processing.

Specific sensory processing characteristics are thought to be genetic traits, which are likely impacted by learning opportunities across contexts and throughout development. In a recent literature review, Homberg, Schubert, Asan, and Aron (2016) discussed evidence related to the genetic bases of high sensitivity. Drawing from the work of Aron, Aron, and Jagiellowicz (2012), the authors argued that sensory sensitivity is partially an evolutionary product of certain people responding more to environmental cues. Strengths of such sensory sensitivity include a deep processing of sensory information and great awareness of environmental subtleties. Other strengths of sensitivity include the underlying cognitive processes that may make individuals pause. For example, Davies, Cicchetti, Hentges, and Sturge-Apple (2013) found that sensitivity may be an adaptive behavior in a negative social environment because individuals are more likely to pick up subtle cues and show behavioral inhibition. However, because these individuals likely have a deeper processing of emotions, sensory sensitivity is also associated with the risk of anxiety and depression (Liss, Timmel, Baxley, & Killingsworth, 2005).

Conversely, sensory seeking has also been investigated as a biological trait associated with decreased sensory registration (Roussos, Giakoumaki, & Bitsios, 2009). When individuals are not as sensitive to environmental sensory stimuli, they may seek out novel and/or intense sensory experiences to increase arousal. Therefore, research suggests that individuals with sensory-seeking traits are more likely to show curiosity and a willingness to try new experiences. Zuckerman (1971) has investigated how high sensation seekers focus on the quest for new, adventurous, and thrill-inducing experiences. Research on thrill and adventure seeking has shown that people with this sensory pattern make decisions in every part of their lives that reflect this need for high-intensity input (Munsey, 2006). When new stimuli are available to high seekers, their orienting reflex moves attention toward the new stimuli.

Studies suggest a developmental course to the maturation and integration of sensory processing, and behavioral and neurophysiological measures indicate there is also developmental course to multisensory integration (i.e., the extent to which individuals are able to coordinate and organize sensory input from multiple modalities). Infant brains prefer synchronous sensory input (e.g., the binding of visual and auditory sensory information; Hyde, Jones, Flom, & Porter, 2011), and such auditory-visual integration begins early in development (Taga, Watanabe, & Homae, 2011). Although auditory-visual integration occurs early, one study showed that novel auditory stimuli slowed infants' ability to process visual information (Robinson & Sloutsky, 2007). Additionally, the integration of looking behaviors begins to integrate with audiovisual behaviors early in development (Hollich & Prince, 2009; Kushnerenko et al., 2013). Studies have found sensory processing differences among preterm infants, showing sensory integration and motor differences compared with those born term even up to 2 years old (Allin et al., 2006; Rahkonen et al., 2013). Related to speech development, lip movements in young infants provide sensorimotor input that contributes to speech production (Yeung & Werker, 2013) and selective attention (Sanders, Stevens, Coch, & Neville, 2006). Most children approximate multisensory patterns of adults during middle childhood to early adolescence (Brandwein et al., 2011; Kedmy, Topper, Cohen-Mimran, & Banai, 2013).

When the developmental course of the integration of sensory information is disrupt-ed, children may have difficulties in certain areas of occupation. There have been studies of children with language impairments, ASD, ADHD, Fragile X syndrome, and other perceptual and brain-related conditions to examine the impact of sensory processing on their adaptive behavior. Generally, findings indicate that when there are competing sensory inputs (e.g., auditory-visual, complex auditory, or visual), children have less tem-poral organization, attention, and timing and communication is harder (Heim, Fried-man, Keil, & Benasich, 2011; Marler & Champlin, 2005; Russo et al., 2010; Stevenson et al., 2014). Other studies suggest that children with conditions show slower processing, suggesting inefficient inhibition (Orekhova et al., 2008) or may have differences in auto-nomic reactions (Schaaf et al., 2010). Children with ASD show strengths in processing simple auditory stimuli such as pure tones (Bonnel et al., 2003) but difficulties in pro-cessing complex auditory input, which may provide insight into the language difficulties in ASD (Jansson-Verkasalo et al., 2003; Teder-Sälejärvi, Pierce, Courchesne, & Hillyard, 2005). Children with Williams syndrome experience visual neural activation with music and other auditory stimuli; such neural confusion between sensory systems likely con-tributes to how they experience challenges in adaptive behaviors (Thornton-Wells et al., 2010).

Interventions to Support Adaptation From a Sensory Processing Perspective

In the following section, we discuss evidence of interventions that support occupa-tional adaptation from a sensory processing perspective. The goal of occupational therapy intervention should be to maximize engagement and participation in everyday activities. In the context of occupational adaptation, interventions should promote development and use of strategies that allow an individual to best meet and negotiate the demands of his or her contexts and environments to successfully participate. Interventions must con-sider the individual's sensory processing patterns as well as the environmental and social supports that match sensory processing patterns. Within each section, we will define and describe each intervention and provide an overview of the studies that have tested the efficacy of that particular intervention.

Environment-Focused Interventions

Environmental modifications may be made in response to children's sensory aversions and preferences. Examples of environment focused interventions to match sensory processing include the use of therapy balls in the classroom, changing the overall classroom environment, and using visual schedules. Kinnealy et al. (2012) tested the effects of changing the lighting and sound in a classroom for children with ASD and showed positive effects on engagement behavior. In this study, the students with ASD preferred halogen lighting and sound-absorbing walls, and they expressed increased focus and comfort in the classroom. Bagatell, Mirigliani, Patterson, Reyes, and Test (2010) tested the impact of sitting on therapy balls in the classroom for children with ASD 5 to 7 years old. Children with high seeking behaviors showed a positive change in behaviors; however, children with poor postural stability were less engaged when sitting on the ball. The literature on visual schedules is extensive (Lequia, Machalicek, & Rispoli, 2012) and shows overall positive effects. When children have pictures to sequentially depict activities and offer them control, they show decreased problem behavior and increased engagement. Given the strengths in visual processing among children with ASD, evidence points to the positive effects of using visual schedules (Case-Smith & Arbesman, 2008).

Interventions Focused on Collaborating With Families

Coaching and parent-mediated interventions directly involve caregivers of children to either create or follow specific behavioral strategies in children's natural environments. This category of intervention models does not necessarily target children's sensory processing; instead, occupational therapists who use these models use their knowledge of how sensory processing knowledge can impact children's participation. Occupational therapists then work with caregivers to figure out how to best design activities to promote child engagement while matching children's sensory preferences and aversions. Overall, this category of interventions helps facilitate family adaptation by promoting a match between child characteristics and environmental factors.

Evidence on coaching and parent-mediated interventions that incorporate sensory processing knowledge has shown promising findings. Occupational performance coaching, which encourages parents to create and implement their own strategies during everyday routines, has been shown to positively impact child participation and parent efficacy among families of children with ASD (Dunn, Cox, Foster, Mische-Lawson, & Tanquary, 2012; Little, Pope, Wallisch, & Dunn, 2018). In another study, Baranek et al. (2015) found that Adapted Responsive Teaching, which promotes parent responsivity in the context of daily activities, positively impacted child sensory responsiveness as well as child adaptive and cognitive skills for children at risk for ASD as compared with a control group. Other parent (Farmer & Reupert, 2013) and adolescent (Edgington, Hill, & Pellicano, 2016) training programs that promote sensory processing knowledge and teach strategies have shown positive outcomes.

Table 7-1

Sensory Processing and the Environment Mismatch and Strategies		
Type	What Might a Mismatch Between Sensory and Environment Look Like?	What Are Strategies to Promote Occupational Adaptation?
Bystander	May appear passive, lethargic, or uninterested. Because he or she is missing cues, the Bystander may appear to miss details.	Take movement breaks throughout the day; use bright-colored paper, sticky notes, or highlighting to draw attention to details or tasks; use a bright visual schedule to attend to details of tasks
Seeker	May appear unfocused, fidgety, constantly moving, messy, and/or a risk taker. Because the Seeker needs increased sensory input to stay focused, he or she may appear busy and inattentive.	Structure activities to include multi-tasking; complete tasks in busy, bright, or noisy environments; use a chair that moves (e.g., with wheels, therapy ball)
Sensor	May appear quiet, uncomfortable, or slightly disengaged. Because the Sensor has a discerning ability to detect sensory information, he or she may appear very particular.	Allow physical space for individual to be at the periphery of the activity; allow time to observe activity before participating; make activity/task predictable or slightly repetitive
Avoider	May appear withdrawn, introverted, or disinterested. Because the Avoider is easily overwhelmed by little sensory input, he or she may appear reserved and nit-picky.	Break up tasks into distinct steps; allow individual time to warm up to activity; give details about the activity/task ahead of time; have individual share control amount of noise, light, movement during activity

The evidence related to environmental modifications and comprehensive approaches such as coaching suggests that the individualized variability of children's sensory processing characteristics must be considered when designing and implementing interventions. Individuals show varying levels of sensory seeking, registration, sensitivities, and avoidances may respond differently to modifications. For example, a bright light or strong scent may be activating for an individual with registration difficulties; however, if a person shows sensory avoidance, the bright light or strong scent may contribute to a mismatch between the task and environment. Instead of conceptualizing sensory processing as solely within the individual, intervention approaches can address the intersection between the person's sensory processing characteristics, the environment, and the occupation. Refer to Tables 7-1 and 7-2 for examples of how specific strategies may contribute to occupational adaptation for individuals with different sensory processing patterns.

Table 7-2

Examples of Adaptations to Support Participation Using Sensory Processing Knowledge				
Sensory Patterns				
Area of Participation	Seekers	Avoiders	Sensors	Bystanders
Daily life	Add more events into an already-busy schedule	Set strong routines for getting ready, managing the day	Create a leisurely plan for morning routine	Design multiple methods for awakening
	Talk with body language and gestures	Follow weekly plan for outfits and meals	Plan quiet spaces for organizing and planning life activities	Create spaces for organizing supplies
	Change paths around town regularly	Shop online for essentials	Find separate places to converse in busy contexts	Set reminders for tasks throughout the day
Work	Select projects requiring creative thinking	Take leadership to provide structure and organization for projects	Focus on work spaces you have control over	Design strategies for reminding you of meeting times, deadlines
	Partner with others to create timelines for projects	Work remotely when possible	Design plan for getting away when overwhelmed (get a drink, take a walk)	Select work teams with high interaction patterns
Dining & eating	Experiment with recipes	Follow a weekly menu	Request changes to food at restaurants	Dine with lively people
	Select active dining experiences	Find ways to eat alone	Follow recipes exactly	Forget ingredients in recipes when cooking
Dressing	Select bright colors, high contrasts, varied textures in clothing	Create wardrobe with only acceptable clothing items	Get clothing items tailored to fit perfectly	Design outfits to make getting ready easier

Adapted from Dunn, W. (2007). *Living sensationally: Understanding your senses.* London, England: Jessica Kingsley Publishers.

ADVANCING KNOWLEDGE ON OCCUPATIONAL ADAPTATION

Sensory processing is a fundamental human experience that provides the information to engage in everyday life. When adaptation is compromised, one possible factor can be related to sensory processing information or interpretation. By addressing the impact of sensory processing on everyday interactions, we can increase adaptive ability. When we conceptualize sensory processing as a one-person factor that impacts how an individual performs across differing environments and occupations, we can move beyond thinking of sensory processing as dysfunction.

To advance knowledge about how sensory processing contributes to occupational adaptation, research and practice must focus on participation. Occupational adaptation is the experiential process by which individuals perform within their everyday environments (Gilfoyle et al., 1981). When there is a mismatch between the environment, the occupation, and the individual's sensory processing characteristics, occupational adaptation is limited. When research and practice focus on participation, we can better understand how sensory processing interacts with environments to impact individuals' performance.

SUMMARY AND IMPLICATIONS

- Sensory processing is a fundamental feature of the human experience that informs us about our bodies and the world around us.

- Drawing from neuroscience literature, research shows that there is variability in how individuals sense and respond differently to sensory information in their environments.

- When persons receive different sensory input or interpret sensory input differently, those persons' behaviors will reflect those differences.

- When persons respond based on the sensory experiences they are having, we might call this their adaptive response, although the behaviors may not be useful in context.

- We support persons' adaptation by informing them, their families and friends, and other providers the characteristics of their sensory patterns so they can explore how those patterns impact everyday life.

REFERENCES

Allin, M., Rooney, M., Griffiths, T., Cuddy, M., Wyatt, J., Rifkin, L., & Murray, R. (2006). Neurological abnormalities in young adults born preterm. *Journal of Neurology, Neurosurgery & Psychiatry, 77*(4), 495-499. doi:10.1136/jnnp.2005.075465

Aron, E. N., Aron, A., & Jagiellowicz, J. (2012). Sensory processing sensitivity: A review in the light of the evolution of biological responsivity. *Personality and Social Psychology Review, 16*(3), 262-282.

Ausderau, K. K., Furlong, M., Sideris, J., Bulluck, J., Little, L. M., Watson, L. R., ... Baranek, G. T. (2014). Sensory subtypes in children with autism spectrum disorder: latent profile transition analysis using a national survey of sensory features. *Journal of Child Psychology and Psychiatry, 55*(8), 935-44. doi:10.1111/jcpp.12219

Ayres, A. J. (1972). *Sensory integration and learning disorders*. Torrance, CA: Western Psychological Services.

Ayres, A. J. (1976). *Southern California sensory integration tests*. Torrance, CA: Western Psychological Services.

Ayres, A.J. (1989). *The sensory integration and praxis tests*. Los Angeles, CA: Western Psychological Services.

Bagatell, N., Mirigliani, G., Patterson, C., Reyes, Y., & Test, L. (2010). Effectiveness of therapy ball chairs on classroom participation in children with autism spectrum disorders. *American Journal of Occupational Therapy, 64*(6), 895-903.

Bagby, M. S., Dickie, V. A., & Baranek, G. T. (2012). How sensory experiences of children with and without autism affect family occupations. *American Journal of Occupational Therapy, 66*(1), 78-86.

Baker, A. E., Lane, A., Angley, M. T., & Young, R. L. (2008). The relationship between sensory processing patterns and behavioural responsiveness in autistic disorder: A pilot study. *Journal of Autism and Developmental Disorders, 38*(5), 867-875.

Baranek, G. T. (2009). *Sensory experiences questionnaire version 3.0*. Unpublished manuscript.

Baranek, G. T., Boyd, B. A., Poe, M. D., David, F. J., & Watson, L. R. (2007). Hyperresponsive sensory patterns in young children with autism, developmental delay, and typical development. *American Journal of Mental Retardation, 112*(4), 233-245.

Baranek, G. T., Little, L. M., Parham, L. D., Ausderau, K. K., & Sabatos-DeVito, M. G. (2014). Sensory features in autism spectrum disorders. In F. R. Volkmar, R. Paul, S. J. Rogers, & K. A. Pelphrey (Eds.), *Handbook of autism and pervasive developmental disorders* (4th ed., Vol. 1, pp. 378-408). Hoboken, NJ: John Wiley & Sons, Inc.

Baranek, G. T., Watson, L. R., Turner-Brown, L., Field, S. H., Crais, E. R., Wakeford, L., … Reznick, J. S. (2015). Preliminary efficacy of adapted responsive teaching for infants at risk of autism spectrum disorder in a community sample. *Autism Research and Treatment, 2015*, 386951. doi:10.1155/2015/386951

Ben-Sasson, A., Cermak, S. A., Orsmond, G. I., Tager-Flusberg, H., Carter, A. S., Kadlec, M. B., & Dunn, W. (2007). Extreme sensory modulation behaviors in toddlers with autism spectrum disorders. *American Journal of Occupational Therapy, 61*(5), 584-592.

Bonnel, A., Mottron, L., Peretz, I., Trudel, M., Gallun, E., & Bonnel, A. M. (2003). Enhanced pitch sensitivity in individuals with autism: A signal detection analysis. *Journal of Cognitive Neuroscience, 15*(2), 226-235.

Bouvet, L., Mottron, L., Valdois, S., & Donnadieu, S. (2016). Auditory stream segregation in autism spectrum disorder: Benefits and downsides of superior perceptual processes. *Journal of Autism and Developmental Disorders, 46*(5), 1553-1561.

Brandwein, A. B., Foxe, J. J., Russo, N. N., Altschuler, T. S., Gomes, H., & Molholm, S. (2011). The development of audiovisual multisensory integration across childhood and early adolescence: A high-density electrical mapping study. *Cerebral Cortex, 21*(5), 1042-1055.

Brown, N. B., & Dunn, W. (2010). Relationship between context and sensory processing in children with autism. *American Journal of Occupational Therapy, 64*(3), 474-483

Carter, A. S., Ben-Sasson, A., & Briggs-Gowan, M. J. (2011). Sensory over-responsivity, psychopathology, and family impairment in school-aged children. *Journal of the American Academy of Child & Adolescent Psychiatry, 50*(12), 1210-1219.

Cascio, C. J., Woynaroski, T., Baranek, G. T., & Wallace, M. T. (2016). Toward an interdisciplinary approach to understanding sensory function in autism spectrum disorder. *Autism Research, 9*(9), 920-925. doi:10.1002/aur.1612

Case-Smith, J., & Arbesman, M. (2008). Evidence-based review of interventions for autism used in or of relevance to occupational therapy. *American Journal of Occupational Therapy, 62*(4), 416-429.

Cheung, P. P., & Siu, A. M. (2009). A comparison of patterns of sensory processing in children with and without developmental disabilities. *Research in Developmental Disabilities, 30*(6), 1468-1480. doi:10.1016/j.ridd.2009.07.009

Cosbey, J., Johnston, S. S., & Dunn, M. L. (2010). Sensory processing disorders and social participation. *American Journal of Occupational Therapy, 64*(3), 462-473.

Davies, P. T., Cicchetti, D., Hentges, R. F., & Sturge-Apple, M. L. (2013). The genetic precursors and the advantageous and disadvantageous sequelae of inhibited temperament: An evolutionary perspective. *Developmental Psychology, 49*(12), 2285-2300.

Dunn, W. (1999). *Sensory profile: User's manual*. San Antonio, TX: Psychological Corporation.

Dunn, W. (2007). *Living sensationally: Understanding your senses*. London, England: Jessica Kingsley Publishers.

Dunn, W. (2014). *Sensory Profile 2: User's manual*. Bloomington, MN: Psychological Corporation.

Dunn, W., & Bennett, D. (2002). Patterns of sensory processing in children with attention deficit hyperactivity disorder. *OTJR: Occupation, Participation and Health, 22*(1), 4-15.

Dunn, W., Cox, J., Foster, L., Mische-Lawson, L., & Tanquary, J. (2012). Impact of a contextual intervention on child participation and parent competence among children with autism spectrum disorders: A pretest–posttest repeated-measures design. *American Journal of Occupational Therapy, 66*(5), 520-528.

Dunn, W., Dean, E., Little, L. M., & Tomchek, S. D. (2018). *Prevalence of sensory processing patterns in a sample of children with and without conditions*. Manuscript submitted for publication.

Dunn, W., Little, L., Dean, E., Robertson, S., & Evans, B. (2016). The state of the science on sensory factors and their impact on daily life for children: A scoping review. *OTJR: Occupation, Participation and Health, 36*(Suppl. 2), 3S.

Dunst, C. J., Bruder, M. B., Trivette, C. M., Hamby, D., Raab, M., & McLean, M. (2001). Characteristics and consequences of everyday natural learning opportunities. *Topics in Early Childhood Special Education, 21*(2), 68-92.

Edgington, L., Hill, V., & Pellicano, E. (2016). The design and implementation of a CBT-based intervention for sensory processing difficulties in adolescents on the autism spectrum. *Research in Developmental Disabilities, 59*, 221-233.

Farmer, J., & Reupert, A. (2013). Understanding autism and understanding my child with autism: An evaluation of a group parent education program in rural Australia. *Australian Journal of Rural Health, 21*(1), 20-27.

Farrow, C. V., & Coulthard, H. (2012). Relationships between sensory sensitivity, anxiety and selective eating in children. *Appetite, 58*(3), 842-846.

Gilfoyle, E., Grady, A., & Moore, J. (1981). *Children adapt* (2nd ed.). Thorofare, NJ: SLACK Incorporated.

Grandin, T., & Scariano, M. M. (1986). *Emergence: Labeled autistic*. Novato, CA: Arena Press.

Heim, S., Friedman, J. T., Keil, A., & Benasich, A. A. (2011). Reduced sensory oscillatory activity during rapid auditory processing as a correlate of language-learning impairment. *Journal of Neurolinguistics, 24*(5), 538-555.

Hilton, C., Graver, K., & LaVesser, P. (2007). Relationship between social competence and sensory processing in children with high functioning autism spectrum disorders. *Research in Autism Spectrum Disorders, 1*(2), 164-173.

Hochhauser, M., & Engel-Yeger, B. (2010). Sensory processing abilities and their relation to participation in leisure activities among children with high-functioning autism spectrum disorder (HFASD). *Research in Autism Spectrum Disorders, 4*(4), 746-754.

Hollich, G., & Prince, C. G. (2009). Comparing infants' preference for correlated audiovisual speech with signal-level computational models. *Developmental Science, 12*(3), 379-387.

Homberg, J. R., Schubert, D., Asan, E., & Aron, E. N. (2016). Sensory processing sensitivity and serotonin gene variance: Insights into mechanisms shaping environmental sensitivity. *Neuroscience & Biobehavioral Reviews, 71*, 472-483. doi:10.1016/j.neubiorev.2016.09.029

Humphry, R., & Wakeford, L. (2008). Development of everyday activities: A model for occupation-centered therapy. *Infants & Young Children, 21*(3), 230-240.

Hyde, D. C., Jones, B. L., Flom, R., & Porter, C. L. (2011). Neural signatures of face-voice synchrony in 5-month-old human infants. *Developmental Psychobiology, 53*(4), 359-370. doi:10.1002/dev.20525

Jansson-Verkasalo, E., Ceponiene, R., Kielinen, M., Suominen, K., Jäntti, V., Linna, S. L., ... Näätänen, R. (2003). Deficient auditory processing in children with Asperger syndrome, as indexed by event-related potentials. *Neuroscience Letters, 338*(3), 197-200.

Jasmin, E., Couture, M., McKinley, P., Reid, G., Fombonne, E., & Gisel, E. (2009). Sensori-motor and daily living skills of preschool children with autism spectrum disorders. *Journal of Autism and Developmental Disorders, 39*(2), 231-241. doi:10.1007/s10803-008-0617-z

Jirikowic, T., Olson, H. C., & Kartin, D. (2008). Sensory processing, school performance, and adaptive behavior of young school-age children with fetal alcohol spectrum disorders. *Physical & Occupational Therapy in Pediatrics, 28*(2), 117-136.

Kedmy, M., Topper, T., Cohen-Mimran, R., & Banai, K. (2013). The development of speech-in-noise perception in Hebrew-speaking school-age children. *Journal of Basic Clinical Physiology and Pharmacology, 24*(3), 185-189. doi:10.1515/jbcpp-2013-0055

King, L. J. (1974). A sensory-integrative approach to schizophrenia. *American Journal of Occupational Therapy, 28*(9), 529-536.

King, L. J. (1987). A sensory-integrative approach to the education of the autistic child. *Occupational Therapy in Health Care, 4*(2), 77-85.

Kinnealey, M., Pfeiffer, B., Miller, J., Roan, C., Shoener, R., & Ellner, M. L. (2012). Effect of classroom modification on attention and engagement of students with autism or dyspraxia. *American Journal of Occupational Therapy, 66*(5), 511-519.

Kushnerenko, E., Tomalski, P., Ballieux, H., Ribeiro, H., Potton, A., Axelsson, E. L., ... Moore, D. G. (2013). Brain responses to audiovisual speech mismatch in infants are associated with individual differences in looking behaviour. *European Journal of Neuroscience, 38*(9), 3363-3369.

Lane, A. E., Molloy, C. A., & Bishop, S. L. (2014). Classification of children with autism spectrum disorder by sensory subtype: A case for sensory-based phenotypes. *Autism Research, 7*(3), 322-333. doi:10.1002/aur.1368

Lequia, J., Machalicek, W., & Rispoli, M. J. (2012). Effects of activity schedules on challenging behavior exhibited in children with autism spectrum disorders: a systematic review. *Research in Autism Spectrum Disorders, 6*(1), 480-492.

Liss, M., Saulnier, C., Fein, D., & Kinsbourne, M. (2006). Sensory and attention abnormalities in autistic spectrum disorders. *Autism, 10*(2), 155-172.

Liss, M., Timmel, L., Baxley, K., & Killingsworth, P. (2005). Sensory processing sensitivity and its relation to parental bonding, anxiety, and depression. *Personality and Individual Differences, 39*(8), 1429-1439.

Little, L. M., Ausderau, K., Sideris, J., & Baranek, G. T. (2015). Activity participation and sensory features among children with autism spectrum disorders. *Journal of Autism and Developmental Disorders, 45*(9), 2981-2990.

Little, L. M., Pope, E., Wallisch, A., & Dunn, W. (2018). Occupational performance coaching via telehealth for families of young children with autism spectrum disorders. *American Journal of Occupational Therapy, 72*(2), 7202205020p1-7202205020p7.

Marler, J. A., & Champlin, C. A. (2005). Sensory processing of backward-masking signals in children with language-learning impairment as assessed with the auditory brainstem response. *Journal of Speech Language Hearing Research, 48*(1), 189-203.

Miller, L. J., Anzalone, M. E., Lane, S., Cermak, S. A., & Osten, E. (2007). Concept evolution in sensory integration: A proposed nosology for diagnosis. *American Journal of Occupational Therapy, 61*(2), 135-140.

Munsey, C. (2006). Frisky, but more risky. *Monitor on Psychology, 37*(7). Retrieved from http://www.apa.org/monitor/julaug06/frisky.aspx

Nadon, G., Feldman, D. E., Dunn, W., & Gisel, E. (2011). Association of sensory processing and eating problems in children with autism spectrum disorders. *Autism Research and Treatment, 2011*. doi:10.1155/2011/541926

Orekhova, E. V., Stroganova, T. A., Prokofyev, A. O., Nygren, G., Gillberg, C., & Elam, M. (2008). Sensory gating in young children with autism: relation to age, IQ, and EEG gamma oscillations. *Neuroscience Letters, 434*(2), 218-223. doi:10.1016/j.neulet.2008.01.066

Orsmond, G. I., & Kuo, H.-Y. (2011). The daily lives of adolescents with an autism spectrum disorder Discretionary time use and activity partners. *Autism, 15*(5), 579-599.

Parham, L. D., & Ecker, C. (2007). *Sensory processing measure (SPM).* Torrance, CA: Western Psychological Services.

Pfeiffer, B., Daly, B. P., Nicholls, E. G., & Gullo, D. F. (2015). Assessing sensory processing problems in children with and without attention deficit hyperactivity disorder. *Physical & Occupational Therapy in Pediatrics, 35*(1), 1-12.

Rahkonen, P., Nevalainen, P., Lauronen, L., Pihko, E., Lano, A., Vanhatalo, S., ... Metsäranta, M. (2013). Cortical somatosensory processing measured by magnetoencephalography predicts neurodevelopment in extremely low-gestational-age infants. *Pediatric Research, 73*(6), 763-771. doi:10.1038/pr.2013.46

Reynolds, S., Bendixen, R. M., Lawrence, T., & Lane, S. J. (2011). A pilot study examining activity participation, sensory responsiveness, and competence in children with high functioning autism spectrum disorder. *Journal of Autism and Developmental Disorders, 41*(11), 1496-1506.

Robinson, C. W., & Sloutsky, V. M. (2007). Visual processing speed: Effects of auditory input on visual processing. *Developmental Science, 10*(6), 734-740.

Roussos, P., Giakoumaki, S. G., & Bitsios, P. (2009). Cognitive and emotional processing in high novelty seeking associated with the L-DRD4 genotype. *Neuropsychologia, 47*(7), 1654-1659. doi:10.1016/j.neuropsychologia.2009.02.005

Russo, N., Foxe, J. J., Brandwein, A. B., Altschuler, T., Gomes, H., & Molholm, S. (2010). Multisensory processing in children with autism: High-density electrical mapping of auditory-somatosensory integration. *Autism Research, 3*(5), 253-267.

Sanders, L. D., Stevens, C., Coch, D., & Neville, H. J. (2006). Selective auditory attention in 3-to 5-year-old children: An event-related potential study. *Neuropsychologia, 44*(11), 2126-2138.

Schaaf, R. C., Benevides, T., Blanche, E. I., Brett-Green, B. A., Burke, J. P., Cohn, E. S., ... Schoen, S. A. (2010). Parasympathetic functions in children with sensory processing disorder. *Frontiers in Integrative Neuroscience, 4*, 4. doi:10.3389/fnint.2010.00004

Schaaf, R. C., & Lane, A. E. (2015). Toward a best-practice protocol for assessment of sensory features in ASD. *Journal of Autism and Developmental Disorders, 45*(5), 1380-1395. doi:10.1007/s10803-014-2299-z

Schaaf, R. C., Toth-Cohen, S., Johnson, S. L., Outten, G., & Benevides, T. W. (2011). The everyday routines of families of children with autism: examining the impact of sensory processing difficulties on the family. *Autism, 15*(3), 373-389. doi:10.1177/1362361310386505

Schkade, J. K., & Schultz, S. (1992). Occupational adaptation: Toward a holistic approach for contemporary practice, part 1. *American Journal of Occupational Therapy, 46*(9), 829-837.

Shochat, T., Tzischinsky, O., & Engel-Yeger, B. (2009). Sensory hypersensitivity as a contributing factor in the relation between sleep and behavioral disorders in normal schoolchildren. *Behavioral Sleep Medicine, 7*(1), 53-62.

Stevenson, R. A., Siemann, J. K., Schneider, B. C., Eberly, H. E., Woynaroski, T. G., Camarata, S. M., & Wallace, M. T. (2014). Multisensory temporal integration in autism spectrum disorders. *Journal of Neuroscience, 34*(3), 691-697. doi:10.1523/jneurosci.3615-13.2014

Taga, G., Watanabe, H., & Homae, F. (2011). Spatiotemporal properties of cortical haemodynamic response to auditory stimuli in sleeping infants revealed by multi-channel near-infrared spectroscopy. *Philosophical Transactions of the Royal Society A: Mathematical, Physical and Engineering Sciences, 369*(1955), 4495-4511. doi:10.1098/rsta.2011.0238

Teder-Sälejärvi, W., Pierce, K., Courchesne, E., & Hillyard, S. (2005). Auditory spatial localization and attention deficits in autistic adults. *Cognitive Brain Research, 23*, 221-234. doi:10.1016/j.cogbrainres.2004.10.021

Thornton-Wells, T. A., Cannistraci, C. J., Anderson, A. W., Kim, C. Y., Eapen, M., Gore, J. C., ... Dykens, E. M. (2010). Auditory attraction: activation of visual cortex by music and sound in Williams syndrome. *American Journal of Intellectual and Developmental Disabilities, 115*(2), 172-189. doi:10.1352/1944-7588-115.172

Watson, L. R., Patten, E., Baranek, G. T., Poe, M., Boyd, B. A., Freuler, A., & Lorenzi, J. (2011). Differential associations between sensory response patterns and language, social, and communication measures in children with autism or other developmental disabilities. *Journal of Speech, Language, and Hearing Research, 54*(6), 1562-1576.

Yeung, H. H., & Werker, J. F. (2013). Lip movements affect infants' audiovisual speech perception. *Psychological Science, 24*(5), 603-612.

Yochman, A., Parush, S., & Ornoy, A. (2004). Responses of preschool children with and without ADHD to sensory events in daily life. *American Journal of Occupational Therapy, 58*(3), 294-302.

Zuckerman, M. (1971). Dimensions of sensation seeking. *Journal of Consulting and Clinical Psychology, 36*(2), 45-52.

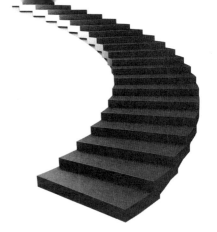

8

Adaptation as a Transaction With the Environment

Perspectives From the Ecology of Human Performance Model

Evan E. Dean, PhD, OTR; Anna Wallisch, PhD, OTR/L; and Winifred Dunn, PhD, OTR, FAOTA

OVERVIEW In this chapter, occupational adaptation is defined as a transactional process through which person and environment are both changed through participation in everyday life. A person is enmeshed in his or her environment, and, through participation, both are changed. This chapter focuses on an ecological model of occupational therapy that uniquely describes how the range of participation in everyday tasks (occupations) is facilitated or hindered by the transaction between the person, the environment, and various features of the task. Within this unique process, occupational adaptation occurs.

Grajo LC, Boisselle AK, eds.
Adaptation Through Occupation:
Multidimensional Perspectives (pp 141-155).
© 2019 SLACK Incorporated.

CHAPTER OBJECTIVES By the end of this chapter, the reader will be able to:
- Describe the ways that person, context, and task features interact to determine a person's participation range.
- Design interventions that address different aspects of the ecological model and a person's adaptation.
- Identify aspects of the context and tasks that affect a person's performance.

QUESTIONS FOR DISCUSSION AND REFLECTION As the reader explores this chapter, let the following questions guide discussion and reflection:
- How can I describe to clients and families how the transactional process between person, occupation, and environment influences occupational participation?
- How can I articulate the relationship between the occupational adaptation process and the person's range of participation in occupations?

INTRODUCTION

Adaptation is generally considered a process through which a person changes as a result of an interaction with the environment. Although this view of adaptation is true, ecological theories maintain that this is not the whole story. Ecological theories of performance (e.g., the Ecology of Human Performance [EHP]) propose that it is impossible to consider a person outside of that person's context. Through an ecological lens, adaptation occurs as a transaction between the person and the context. For example, a young adult may thrive in a small classroom where the teacher has time for individual instruction. In this environment, the student believes he is a good student and performs as a good student. Yet, the student may struggle in a large classroom with a lot of distractions. If the student's daily experience involves large, distracting classrooms, the student then has the option of developing new strategies to successfully engage in the new environment, talk with the teacher or other professionals to create an atmosphere more conducive to learning, or conclude that he is not a good student and quit trying.

EHP, which describes human performance within the general population, provides a strong framework for considering adaptation from an ecological lens. Additionally, EHP offers intervention strategies so that professionals can choose whether to focus on the person, tasks, or environments. As we think about how people live everyday life, we realize everyone learns new skills, makes adjustments, and finds better fitting contexts to meet his or her own needs. Moving forward, occupational therapy must consider the entirety of adaptation processes for everyone, not just those with specified conditions.

EHP was designed by the Department of Occupational Therapy Education at the University of Kansas. The purpose was to create a conceptual framework for the research efforts of the department, guide curriculum development for their entry-level occupational therapy program, and create a model for interdisciplinary collaborations. EHP was based on research from ecological psychology, child development, and developmental psychology (Bronfenbrenner, 1979; Bruner, 1989). It describes the role of context in participation and adaptation.

In this chapter, we will explore the basic assumptions, core constructs, and relationships between the core concepts of EHP. From an ecological perspective, it is through the relationships among the core constructs that adaptation occurs. We will also describe how intervention options emerge from the core ideas and illustrate EHP in a practice context through a case study.

Basic Assumptions

Through EHP, the person and the environment both adapt through participation in daily life. This section will outline the basic assumptions of the EHP model and further highlight the connection between person and context.

Persons and Their Contexts Are Dynamic and Interacting

1. *It is impossible to understand the person without also understanding the person's context.* People may not fully understand the complexities of human behaviors and performance until we analyze contextual features. Context provides a means to facilitate and support an individual's performance and can also make performance more challenging, so without contextual information, performance data are incomplete (Dunn, Brown, & Youngstrom, 2003).

2. *Persons influence contexts, and contexts influence persons.* The relationship between the person and context is ever changing. Different contexts afford individuals different performance patterns; conversely, different skills and abilities allow for us to display different performance patterns in differing contexts (Dunn et al., 2003).

3. *A person's performance range is determined by the transaction between the person and the context.* Two individuals with the same condition may present with completely different performance patterns based around additional person factors, contextual features, and the meaningfulness of the tasks to the individual (Dunn et al., 2003). For example, one person may be interested in cooking, so she can adapt to a kitchen in a cabin with only a few tools, creating an expanded performance range. Another person in that same cabin might not have the personal resources or interest in cooking, so she will have a limited ability to adapt in the context, creating a narrower performance range.

Contrived Contexts Differ From Natural Contexts

1. *When compared with natural environments, contrived contexts may not reflect true performance.* Contrived contexts are often set up to elicit certain behaviors and performance patterns; therefore, because the contextual features differ from the natural context, an individual may perform in a differing manner. Contrived contexts are not authentic to the person, and thus may depict true performance outcomes. For instance, an adult with an intellectual disability who is practicing job skills may perform better in a quiet environment with all materials set up for him; however,

when in an authentic job context, the environment may be much louder and set-up cues may not exist, thus changing performance. Alternatively, if a person needs more stimulation to engage in activities, the quiet environment may make the person look less capable than is actually true.

2. *Assessment and intervention best approximate the person's true performance when enacted in natural environments.* Therapists must understand how contrived contexts provide different performance outcomes when compared with authentic contexts, and therefore potentially provide inaccurate observation of a person's abilities. Erroneous assessment information may lead to unnecessary and inapplicable interventions.

3. *Contrived contexts impact the person's ability to adapt to task demands.* A contrived context could provide more resources than one would have in an authentic context, thus changing the adaptation profile. For example, in a rehab setting, the bathroom might already be adapted for those who have had brain injuries. With grab bars and safe surfaces for navigating, the person may be successful at toileting or getting into the shower. Although this is safer, the adapted bathroom context does not afford the opportunity to know how a person might adapt to a bathroom with less supports.

Occupational Therapy Involves the Promotion of Self-Determination and Inclusion of Persons With Disabilities in All Aspects of Society

1. *The occupational therapy process begins when the person and/or family identifies what the person wants or needs.* EHP recognizes the importance of providing a client-centered approach. Individuals are autonomous and act as the decision makers in the therapeutic process. When individuals are actively involved in the process, motivation will likely increase (Dunn, 2007).

2. *Occupational therapy practice includes making changes in systems so that persons with conditions receive the full rights and privileges they are due.* Occupational therapists must advocate for the rights for individuals with disabilities within the community to generate change in society and policy (Dunn et al., 2003). Likewise, occupational therapists may play a pivotal role in expanding the opportunities for individuals with conditions.

Independence Occurs When a Person's Wants and Needs Are Fulfilled

1. *Utilizing the support of other persons or assistive devices does not indicate dependence.* Each individual, regardless of condition, utilizes others or devices to successfully perform a task (Dunn et al., 2003). Frequently, we create reminders on our phones to visually support us with organizing our day or ask a spouse to pick up additional items at the store due to a busy schedule. These supports we use in our daily life are adaptations we make to our environment that allow us to function optimally. Thus, utilizing devices or the assistance of others does not indicate dependence, but indicates resourcefulness (Dunn et al., 2003).

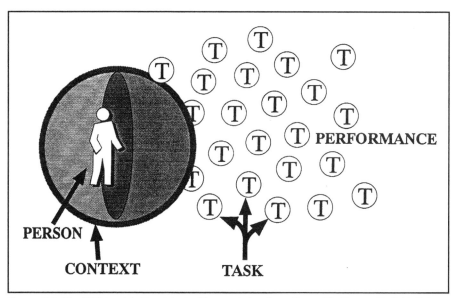

Figure 8-1. The EHP model. (Reprinted with permission from Dunn, W., Brown, C., & McGuigan, A. [1994]. The ecology of human performance: A framework for considering the effect of context. *American Journal of Occupational Therapy, 48*[7], 595-607. doi:10.5014/ajot.48.7.595)

2. *Environmental adjustments can support participation early in the therapeutic process.* Many therapists start by attempting to address and/or fix person factors, and when performance outcomes and goals are not achieved, they resort to contextual interventions (Dunn et al., 2003). However, many times adapting or altering contextual features may provide quicker and more successful performance outcomes (Dunn et al., 2003).

KEY CONSTRUCTS

Four primary constructs provide the foundation for the EHP model: person, task, context, and performance. Together, these constructs illustrate the complex interactions that support or interfere with a person's ability to participate successfully and with satisfaction. The four core constructs are outlined here. Figure 8-1 illustrates the relationships among the key constructs.

Person

EHP provides the means to address each person's individual characteristics, thus providing a client-centered framework (Dunn et al., 2003). EHP characterizes the person as a complex compilation of sensorimotor, cognitive, and psychosocial abilities, as well as personal interests, values, and experiences (Dunn et al., 2003). However, within the EHP framework, the only way to truly see and understand person factors is through analyzing the context surrounding the person (Dunn, Brown, & McGuigan, 1994). This means the context may influence a person's abilities and skills due to different demands within different contexts. For instance, runners may alter their contexts during the hot summer months by using an indoor track (physical context) or running earlier (temporal context) in the morning to decrease contextual demands and maintain successful performance during extreme heat.

Task

EHP defines task as an objective set of behaviors needed to engage in performance to reach a goal (Dunn et al., 2003), and each person has the opportunity to perform a countless number of tasks (Dunn et al., 1994). Additionally, task demands define the behaviors warranted for successful performance.

However, person and context factors define the availability and opportunities to engage in the myriad of tasks (Dunn et al., 2003). For example, making coffee every morning requires the appropriate measurement of coffee grounds and pouring water and coffee. However, task demands and the sequence of steps changes slightly with regard to which coffee device (physical context) you use (e.g., French press, single-serve coffee machines, drip). The device one uses defines the behaviors and skills needed to complete making coffee (e.g., measuring coffee grounds is unnecessary with a single-serve coffee machine that uses pods).

Context

Four contextual features (i.e., the environments) surround the person factors: temporal (including age, life cycle, health status, and expectations related to these aspects), physical (all objects and elements around us), social (our relationships and norms), and cultural environments (beliefs and values; Dunn, 2007). A critical component of EHP relates to the interaction between the person and environment, which influences the behaviors and level of participation possible (Dunn, 2007). For instance, the demands within our home are much different than demands at work, and many of our behaviors change when transitioning between these contexts. In addition, context may either facilitate or act as a barrier to a person's performance on a given task. For example, where a person lives (physical context) may present a barrier to participation if that person wants to enter an occupational therapy program in an area where no program exists. The person may have to move to a new area without family supports or may have to work extra hours to afford out-of-state tuition.

Performance

Performance refers to a person's engagement in tasks within a context. Each person has a given performance range, which refers to the number and types of tasks available to a person, which is determined by the interaction between the person and context factors (Dunn et al., 2003). For instance, one is more likely to show interest in piano playing if a piano is readily available in the home (physical context). In this situation, the context supports participation (practice) and therefore an increased performance range of piano skills. However, one may not show interest to piano playing (person factors) even with the piano available, and therefore may not explore performance with music.

RELATIONSHIP AMONG CONSTRUCTS

A critical and dynamic relationship exists between the person variables and context variables (Dunn, 2007). With each new context, an individual may have the opportunity to develop new skills and abilities due to different demands, and vice versa, where the development of new skills and abilities may allow a person to perform in a different manner when in a given context. For instance, when we transition from renting to owning a home, the context demands change. Many times, we must learn many new skills to maintain our homes (e.g., plumbing, electrical, yard work), and if we do not acquire a given skill within our performance range, we rely on others.

An additional relationship exists with the combination of multiple tasks. As people adapt through participating in new experiences (and gain more expertise through the process), more opportunities for adaptation are available. For example, when we are 16 years old we begin learning how to drive (an occupation), which comprises myriad tasks (e.g., finding the keys, putting the seat belt on, reversing, parking); however, as we gain years of practice, the demands of driving becomes less effortful and instead more automatic and second nature. In this situation, our performance range may expand and include advanced driving tasks such as parallel parking as we continue to participate in the occupation. Therefore, as we engage in driving in new contexts where parallel parking is a demand, we may increase our performance range and adapt to meet the demands of different contexts.

Finally, context presents a range of possibilities for any given situation. We must consider not only a person's skills and abilities, but also what the context makes available to the person to determine the depth and breadth of the performance range. A person trained as a pet groomer may have a wide range of personal skills for grooming many types of dogs and cats, but in a setting in which only small dogs are groomed, the groomer will display a narrower performance range. The performance range includes tasks that are meaningful to an individual and possible because of the characteristics of the context (Dunn et al., 2003).

THERAPEUTIC INTERVENTION

EHP provides five therapeutic interventions to address the dynamic relationship between the person, context, task, and performance variables. Extending the framework to include intervention options makes EHP unique. The interventions include establish/restore, alter, adapt/modify, prevent, and create. These original terms are now part of the common language of occupational therapy (American Occupational Therapy Association, 2014); to demonstrate applicability to the general population, we provide a simple phrase for each intervention below (Table 8-1).

Table 8-1

Common Language Phrases for Ecology of Human Performance Interventions	
EHP Intervention	Common Language for This Intervention
Establish/restore	Learn something new every day
Alter	Find a better place
Adapt/modify	Make it easier to do
Prevent	Think ahead
Create	Make it work for everyone

Establish/Restore: Learn Something New Every Day

The establish/restore intervention strategy focuses on an individual's skills and abilities, and a therapist aims to improve person variables (Dunn et al., 2003). Therapists may either *establish* new skills an individual has not yet learned or *restore* skills lost due to an injury or illness (Dunn et al., 2003). Although establish/restore approaches primarily address person factors, context plays an important role because context provides a means to perform certain tasks (Dunn et al., 1994). With the start to a new school year, we see college students restoring studying strategies and homework routines, as well as establishing new skills from learning new material.

Alter: Find a Better Place

The alter intervention strategy primarily focuses on addressing contextual factors (Dunn, 2007). Therapists must identify contextual features that may support an individual's performance while utilizing a person's current skills and abilities (Dunn et al., 1994). Thus, the therapist does not act to fix or improve upon skills, nor does the therapist make changes to the context; rather, the therapist acts to find a better match between the person and environment for successful performance. For instance, the placement of a washer or dryer within the home may increase performance with laundry. Specifically, if the location of the washer and dryer is changed and placed within closer proximity to bedrooms, the task demands decrease (e.g., less lifting and time spent carrying laundry, no stairs). By simply finding a better place for the washer and dryer rather than changing person factors or task demands, we may facilitate performance in laundry.

Another example of using an alter strategy is finding an optimal study location. A student may find a coffee shop too loud or crowded and may perform better in a library or another quiet place. Another student, however, may find the noisy environment optimal for studying. Each person has unique preferences and will need to find the right fit of study environment. Some students may not have the insight or experience to make these decisions on their own. In these cases, occupational therapists can help them understand their environmental preferences and find places that will support their studying.

Adapt/Modify: Make It Easier to Do

The third intervention strategy allows a therapist to adapt or change the current contextual features and task demands to best support the performance within the frame of a person's skills and abilities (Dunn et al., 1994). For example, many of us search for information online every day; however, with the advancements in technology, there are many ways to make this task easier. Using a keyboard on a computer or on a phone provides two options for adapting the physical contexts to increase performance. Additionally, many phones now have capabilities where you may speak to your phone to search online; therefore, one may adapt the task by eliminating typing demands to make searching online easier to do. These environmental adaptations can also produce adaptation within the individual. The individual can become more confident with using technology and become more productive.

Prevent: Think Ahead

The fourth intervention strategy addresses person, context, and task factors to avert possible future performance problems from developing. Thus, therapists may hypothesize or anticipate negative outcomes and develop strategies by addressing either the person factors, context factors, or task demands to support performance (Dunn, 2007). As an example, it is easy to forget appointments, meetings, or deadlines that do not occur on a regular basis or are outside of one's normal routine. Forgetting these events often results in a negative outcome (e.g., missing details about a project, paying a fee for missing an appointment). One way to think ahead or prevent forgetting an event is to decrease the task demands on one's memory by using sticky notes or calendar alerts as reminders. Individual adaptation occurs when a person uses these strategies on a routine basis and increases his or her efficiency with remembering events.

Create: Make It Work for Everyone

The final intervention strategy focuses more on addressing community and population-based features by creating circumstances and environments that allow optimal performance. Additionally, the create intervention allows therapists to strategize ways to target the person, context, and task to augment performance for a community as a whole (Dunn et al., 2003). Many alter interventions are seen as advantageous for more than one individual, and when disseminated to the general public, this intervention becomes a create approach. Specifically, universal design originates by altering the context for individuals who require the contextual change (e.g., automatic doors, multilevel countertops); however, these changes often prove beneficial for the performance of everyone. For example, adding automatic doors is required for some individuals with wheelchairs, but automatic doors facilitate performance for anyone pushing a grocery cart or stroller, thus creating a context that works for everyone.

ECOLOGY OF HUMAN PERFORMANCE CASE STUDY

Caroline is a 30-year-old woman who sought support from an occupational therapist at her community support agency (CSA) for adults with intellectual disability. The occupational therapist leads the employment program at the CSA, and Caroline wanted a job. The therapist agreed to assess Caroline's personal features and skills (i.e., person and performance factors respectively), morning routine (i.e., tasks), and contextual factors (i.e., environmental) while he helped her look for a job.

> In the following text, we provide comment boxes to mark where the EHP constructs and interventions are occurring in Caroline's story; we also provide a brief rationale for each intervention choice.

Person and Task Factors

The therapist's first consideration was Caroline's person factors. Caroline's support team was concerned about Caroline looking for employment because she came into the CSA with poor personal hygiene and wearing unclean clothes. When visiting Caroline at her home, Caroline and the therapist began with general conversation; during this conversation, the therapist became aware of Caroline's interest in fashion. She had many fashion magazines around her apartment, and she took a special interest in organizing her clothing. Caroline had limited work experience involving periodic volunteering at a food bank and her church.

The therapist began to address Caroline's goals by providing <u>training for Caroline to teach her the importance of hygiene and dressing for employment. Caroline demonstrated she knew how to wash herself and take care of her clothes.</u>

> The therapist starts by providing an ESTABLISH/RESTORE approach with Caroline.

Additionally, the therapist collaborated with Caroline to create a <u>visual schedule to prompt</u> Caroline to complete her morning hygiene routine.

> Here, we see the therapist employing an ADAPT intervention. The therapist adjusts the task demands by providing visual cues in an attempt to facilitate Caroline's morning routine.

Finally, Caroline determined how long it would take to complete the routine and <u>set her alarm to have enough time in the morning to get ready</u>. With these supports in place, Caroline's hygiene remained unchanged.

> Here is an additional ADAPT intervention, where the task demands are adjusted to make success possible for Caroline, e.g., more time is allotted for Caroline's morning routine.

Table 8-2 summarizes person and task features of Caroline's daily routines, which are the factors the person brings to life activities in the EHP framework. Considered from a person standpoint, some of the performance factors seem to be at odds with each other. For example, Caroline keeps her closet neat and her dress clothes are folded nicely, but she generally wears rumpled or dirty clothes during the day. Additionally, she likes to organize her clothes and can do so with little support, indicating a strength in attention to detail; however, she needs frequent prompts to complete her morning routine in a timely manner prior to attending the CSA.

Contextual Features

Considered from a context perspective, however, Caroline's performance features begin to make sense. Table 8-3 summarizes the therapist's impressions of Caroline's context, a key feature of the EHP framework. There is little expectation that people dress nicely at the CSA, and Caroline's options for social interaction outside of the CSA are limited. Therefore, there is little need for Caroline to dress nicely. Considering the cleaning tasks at the agency, Caroline may be bored because she has been doing the same tasks for several years.

When visiting Caroline's home, <u>the therapist noticed that Caroline enjoyed arranging the clothes in her closet</u>, which was in contrast to her daily appearance.

> The therapist begins to understand Caroline's performance range in tasks. This new insight will help when designing the best fit among the person, the tasks, and the context as EHP suggests.

Table 8-2

Caroline's Person and Task Features of Daily Routines			
Person Variables	Activities of Daily Living	Work/Productive Activity	Leisure
Sensorimotor	Caroline gets a lot of satisfaction out of arranging her clothes neatly in her closet.	Caroline helps with chores at home and during the day and particularly enjoys arranging supplies and organizing cupboards.	Caroline prefers interacting with one or two friends at a time; she says large groups are too loud.
Cognitive	Caroline rushes through daily routines and generally skips most of her hygiene.	Caroline needs frequent support to stay on task during cleaning tasks.	Caroline enjoys fashion and nail art, although she often forgets to place caps on nail polish, and her polish dries out or spills.
Psychosocial	Caroline likes to look through fashion magazines and talk to people about clothes.	Caroline likes to interact with visitors at the CSA. She would like a job working in retail.	Caroline typically attends social events with people from the CSA; however, she has expressed that she would like to find other friends.

The therapist asked about the difference, and Caroline discussed her interest in fashion. While attempting to establish the hygiene routine, and based on the conversation about fashion, the therapist worked with Caroline to find and apply for jobs with clothing retailers.

A few weeks later, an employer notified Caroline that they would like to interview her. The following day, which was 3 days before the interview, Caroline came in to the program dressed professionally with her teeth brushed and hair washed.

> The therapist observes Caroline behaving differently as she anticipated entering an authentic context, the retail interview. This change in Caroline's presentation informs the therapist how important authentic opportunities are for truly seeing the person.

The therapist complimented Caroline on her appearance and asked what caused the change. Caroline replied "I have an interview."

Table 8-3

Summary and Analysis of Contextual Features	
Name: Caroline	
C = Contributing factor to participation B = Possible barrier to participation ? = It is unclear how this feature affects participation	Code
Physical	
• Caroline attends a CSA for adults with intellectual disability.	C
• The program provides transportation for Caroline's activities.	C
• Caroline lives in a home with two other women and a caregiver.	?
Social	
• All caregivers and program participants know Caroline.	C
• Caroline spends most of her day at the CSA.	B
• When Caroline accesses the community, she is typically accompanied by five to seven other adults with intellectual disability and at least one caregiver.	B
• Caroline wants a job and would like to spend more time on individual vs group-based pursuits in the community.	C
Cultural	
• Most program participants and caregivers wear loose, comfortable clothes (e.g., baggy shorts, jeans, or sweat pants) at the CSA.	?
• When accessing the community, Caroline has little interaction with people outside of her group.	B
Temporal	
• Caroline is 30 years old.	?
• She has been attending the CSA for 9 years.	?
• Caroline has an intellectual disability (which can affect developmental learning).	?

Performance Features

Caroline continued with her hygiene and dressing routine and eventually found out she got the job at the clothing retailer. She has continued washing and dressing nicely both for her job and when she visits the CSA. In the end, Caroline's context needed to be authentic for her to complete the hygiene routine. When she got the interview, she was no longer a day program member, but a job seeker. The demands associated with her employment context changed, and thus aspects of Caroline's person and task variables changed.

> **For Caroline, being an employee at the retail store working with clothing matched her interests and goals.**

She understood the expectations of being a job seeker and began meeting those expectations. Caroline's performance range expanded as she found opportunities to participate in multiple contexts and employ her person and task skills within areas of her interests.

Advancing the Knowledge on Occupational Adaptation

Adaptation occurs when the environment and tasks match the interests and strengths of the person. This chapter introduced a contextual approach to adaptation. In EHP, persons cannot be considered outside of their contexts. The person, environment, task, and performance are key elements of the model and together describe participation in context. The environment can support or inhibit participation for all people and should be a consideration for intervention. Intervention in EHP can be directed toward the person, the task, or the environment. By directing intervention toward the task or environment, therapists can support participation for individuals and communities. Accessible environments can support participation for all.

Although EHP was designed to bring more attention to focusing intervention on the environment, it is important to consider person factors and task factors simultaneously. That is, to adapt an environment, a therapist also needs to know who will be accessing the environment and what he or she will be doing there. Adapting an environment to meet the sensory preferences of a group will look different from adaptations needed to accommodate physical differences.

SUMMARY AND IMPLICATIONS

- EHP, as an ecological theory, provides new insights into the adaptation process.
- EHP highlights the transactional relationship between the person and the environment, whereby through engagement in occupation, the person and their environment adapt.
- EHP intervention strategies consider how people adapt to task demands and how the environment may be adapted to promote optimal functioning.
- There are times in everyone's life when he or she is more or less successful with adaptation. During these times, occupational therapists may support participation by adapting tasks and environments to meet a person's needs.

REFERENCES

American Occupational Therapy Association. (2014). Occupational Therapy Practice Framework: Domain and Process (3rd ed.). *American Journal of Occupational Therapy, 68*(Suppl. 1), S1-S48. doi:10.5014/ajot.2014.682006

Bronfenbrenner, U. (1979). *The ecology of human development: Experiments by design and nature.* Cambridge, MA: Harvard University Press.

Bruner, J. (1989). *Acts of meaning.* Cambridge, MA: Harvard University Press.

Dunn, W. (2007). Ecology of Human Performance model. In S. Dunbar (Ed.), *Occupational therapy models for intervention with children and families* (pp. 127-156). Thorofare, NJ: SLACK Incorporated.

Dunn, W., Brown, C., & McGuigan, A. (1994). The ecology of human performance: A framework for considering the effect of context. *American Journal of Occupational Therapy, 48*(7), 595-607. doi:10.5014/ajot.48.7.595

Dunn, W., Brown, C., & Youngstrom, M. J. (2003). Ecological model of occupation. In P. Kramer, J. Hinojosa, & C. B. Royeen (Eds.), *Perspectives in human occupation: Participation in life* (pp. 222-263). Baltimore, MD: Lippincott Williams & Wilkins.

Section IV

OCCUPATIONAL ADAPTATION IN OCCUPATIONAL SCIENCE

Lenin C. Grajo, PhD, EdM, OTR/L and Angela K. Boisselle, PhD, OTR, ATP

OVERVIEW

This section focuses on occupational adaptation from an occupational science perspective. Chapter 9 presents a theoretical evolution of the constructs of occupation, adaptation, and participation and how the three constructs relate to each other. In many definitions throughout this book, occupational adaptation is described as a process that emerges from the transaction of the person and the environment. Chapter 9 is distinguished from other chapters in that the *transactional perspective of occupation* is described to propose an understanding of the construct of occupational adaptation as a process that emerges from situations within the evolving relationship between person and environment rather than a person-centered perspective.

Chapter 10 contextualizes many of the theoretical assertions of Chapter 9 by presenting the lived experience of occupational adaptation. Several research studies conducted outside of the United States are presented in the chapter to illustrate and exemplify the process of occupational adaptation as humans experience change, life transitions, and adverse life experiences. In this chapter, several case studies from published research are highlighted to define the evolving nature of the process of occupational adaptation and how occupational adaptation is a universal, culturally relevant construct.

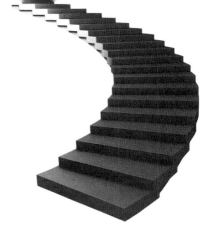

9

An Occupational Science Perspective on Occupation, Adaptation, and Participation

Rebecca M. Aldrich, PhD, OTR/L and
Kendra Heatwole Shank, PhD, OTR/L

OVERVIEW In this chapter, occupational adaptation is defined as planned, provisional, and possible changes enacted through occupations and oriented toward future desired goals of occupational engagement, role fulfillment, or identity development. This chapter illustrates how occupational science, and a transactional perspective in particular, has reframed occupation, adaptation, and participation as processes that hinge on the person-environment relationship. Instead of considering action as occurring on or in an environment, a transactional perspective foregrounds the connectedness of person and environment and moves away from understanding occupational adaptation as a solely individual process. Overall, this chapter suggests that occupational science provides theoretical grounding for understanding occupational adaptation relative to larger issues such as occupational justice.

Grajo LC, Boisselle AK, eds.
Adaptation Through Occupation:
Multidimensional Perspectives (pp 159-174).
© 2019 SLACK Incorporated.

CHAPTER OBJECTIVES By the end of this chapter, the reader will be able to:

- Trace the conceptual development of occupation, adaptation, and participation from their roots in the occupational therapy literature to their current expression in the occupational science literature.
- Summarize how occupational science inquiry has shifted understandings about occupation, adaptation, and participation.
- Articulate how expanded understandings about occupation, adaptation, and participation can influence occupation-focused research and practice, including the pursuit of occupational justice.

QUESTIONS FOR DISCUSSION AND REFLECTION As the reader explores this chapter, let the following questions guide discussion and reflection:

- How will the linkage of participation with health and well-being expand my knowledge of occupational adaptation?
- What factors of the person-environment relationship influence adaptation?

INTRODUCTION

Since the late 1970s, various notions of adaptation have helped occupational therapists think about how humans respond to the environment through action. Wood (1996) argued that the term *adaptation* has been used "to describe processes of skill acquisition, functional outcomes, technological aids, temporal balance of occupations, as well as modifications of how activities are presented, of objects and positioning involved in activities, and of activity environments, including their sociocultural dimensions" (p. 627). Recent scholarship about adaptation and occupation has built on these ideas against the backdrop of occupational science's development. When occupational science was introduced as a formal academic discipline in 1989 (Yerxa, Clark, Jackson, Pierce, & Zemke, 1990), its founders at the University of Southern California outlined two purposes: (1) occupational science should generate knowledge about occupation and humans as occupational beings "without immediate application to therapeutic intervention" (Clark et al., 1991, p. 307), and (2) occupational science should enhance the practice of occupational therapy (Molke, Laliberte Rudman, & Polatajko, 2004; Molineux & Whiteford, 2011; Pierce, 2012). Because occupational science was born within the context of occupational therapy, much of the discipline's conceptual advances have origins in occupational therapy's ideas; however, public health, anthropology, sociology, psychology, and other fields have subsequently shaped occupational science's trajectory and taken the discipline's understandings in new directions.

In an early occupational science publication, Frank (1996) argued that "occupational science will need to go beyond the definitions of adaptation that occupational therapists have insightfully developed" because of the discipline's concern with "moral agency" (p. 50). Increasing emphases on population-level issues related to social inclusion and justice (Whiteford & Hocking, 2012) illustrate how occupational science's moral commitments (Frank, 2012) have furthered thinking on ideas about occupation and adaptation in ways that might not have occurred in occupational therapy alone. In the following pages, we provide an overview of the conceptual development of occupation, adaptation, and a related term, *participation*, to highlight how occupational science has expanded on occupational therapy's foundation in those domains. We then discuss the implications of these expansions and suggest that a stronger theoretical grounding of ideas about occupation, adaptation, and participation creates spaces for broader inquiries about problematic situations such as occupational injustices.

DEVELOPMENT OF CONCEPTS

Occupation

The concept of *occupation* and its espoused relation to human health is the glue that binds occupational science to occupational therapy. From the founding of occupational therapy through the present time, scholars have worked to hone their understandings about occupation and synthesize their knowledge into a comprehensive yet comprehensible central concept. As Laliberte Rudman and Aldrich (2017) noted, it can be tricky to reconcile the many definitions of occupation that exist. Since the inception of occupational therapy, many scholars (Christiansen, 1994; Royeen, 2002) have attempted to elucidate and elaborate occupation as the "active or 'doing' process of a person engaged in goal-directed, intrinsically gratifying, and culturally appropriate activity" (Evans, 1987, p. 627). In 1995, an American Occupational Therapy Association (AOTA) position paper compiled various definitions of occupation and framed it as "the ordinary and familiar things people do every day" that are "organizing, self-fulfilling" and "an important mechanism of adaptation" (Christiansen, Clark, Kielhofner, Rogers, & Nelson, 1995, p. 1015). This position paper, along with Schwartz's (2003) historical review of occupation, traced several definitional elements back to occupational therapy founders such as Adolf Meyer, William Rush Dunton, Eleanor Clarke Slagle, and Susan Johnson. These founders justified the need for a new profession—occupational therapy—in part by noting the benefits of occupation for recovery and adaptation "to the problems of living" (Hinojosa, Kramer, Royeen, & Luebben, 2003, p. 26). They also "embraced the recognition that an individual's health was bound up in the intricacies of daily experiences in a complex physical and social world" (Kielhofner & Burke, 1977, p. 679). Thus, from the early days of the profession, adaptation and individualized experience were seen as defining features of occupation (Hinojosa et al., 2003).

In the second half of the 20th century, as scholars recognized "the lack of a science unique to occupation" (Hinojosa et al., 2003, p. 29) and began in earnest to develop occupational science (Clark et al., 1991), *general systems theory* (von Bertalanffy, 1962) arose as a preferred way of explaining occupational behavior. With roots in mathematics and physical sciences (Byrne, 1998), general systems theory reinforced the linear understandings of occupation and adaptation (Aldrich, 2008) that had origins in psychology's stimulus-response behaviorist models. Systems-based explanations of occupation remained dominant throughout the 1980s (Kielhofner & Burke, 1980) and 1990s (Gray, Kennedy, & Zemke, 1996a, 1996b) as a basis for describing how complex, dynamic occupations occur in environments (Wu & Lin, 1999). During this time, occupational science continued its focus on occupation "as a type of activity which involves some sort of participation by the individual" (Gray, 1997, p. 9), and attempts to differentiate between occupation and activity (Golledge, 1998; Pierce, 2001) reinforced individual meaning and subjective experience as defining features of occupation.

By the 2000s, critiques of systems theories began to emerge as scholars acknowledged that "simple explanations of occupation may misinform and limit the development of the field of occupational science" (Occupational Terminology, 2001, p. 38). These critiques reflected a larger transition to viewing knowledge as situated and pluralistic instead of universal and singular. Whiteford, Townsend, and Hocking (2000) argued that such a view, which was rooted in postmodernism, influenced occupational science's aim "to challenge the privileging of one group or perspective over another, and to illuminate the diverse perspectives, temporality, and situatedness of occupation in its cultural, physical, social, and institutional context" (p. 66). Such an aim was becoming evident in occupational scientists' suggestions that systems theories were inadequate bases for describing occupation and adaptation. For example, Cutchin (2004) highlighted the problems inherent in dynamic systems theory's understanding of the environment as a container of human action, and Eakman (2007) noted that applications of systems theories reinforced a focus on individual systems at the expense of social systems.

The view of occupation as an individualized phenomenon has been a primary point of discussion in occupational science during the first two decades of the 2000s. Dickie, Cutchin, and Humphry noted in 2006, "it is neither surprising, nor unreasonable that occupational science would describe occupation as individualistic and health focused, given [that]…much of occupational therapy takes place in health care or educational settings where the individual is the focus of concern" (p. 84). They argued, however, that a focus on individuals was insufficient for fully conceptualizing occupation. Building on Cutchin's (2004) earlier critiques of systems theories and their dualistic separation of person and environment, Dickie, Cutchin, and Humphry (2006) proposed that occupations must be understood as *transactions* that reflect the interpenetration and connectedness of person and environment. Grounded in John Dewey's philosophy, this assertion represented a dramatic shift away from conceptualizations of occupation as "action on the environment [that requires] the interaction of an active human being with a particular environmental context" (Henderson, 1996, p. 421). Scholars who have since taken up a transactional perspective of occupation have moved to describing occupation as "a type of relational action through which habit, context, and creativity are coordinated toward a provisional yet particular meaningful outcome that is always in process" (Cutchin, Aldrich, Bailliard, & Coppola, 2008, p. 164). Cutchin and Dickie's (2013) book, along with several articles in the *Journal of Occupational Science*, offers an array of examples of how this perspective is being taken up and expanded by scholars who are concerned with occupation.

Following Dickie, Cutchin, and Humphry's lead, many occupational scientists have begun to highlight occupation as a social phenomenon where individual experiences are seen as situated within socially generated value systems and structures (Laliberte Rudman, 2013). In an effort to transcend a primary focus on individuals, occupational scientists have also advocated shifting from understanding the *experience* of occupation to understanding the phenomenon of occupation itself. Wright-St. Clair, Hocking, Bunrayong, Vittayakorn, and Rattakorn's (2005) exploration of meal preparation and

Dickie's (2003) explorations of quilt making are two examples of studies that focus on understanding occupation itself. To further this effort, Hocking (2009) outlined 14 parameters (e.g., rules, norms, outcomes, personal and cultural meanings, economic and historical contexts) to organize descriptions of and research on occupation, and Dickie (2010) exemplified how occupations such as pottery making could be analyzed as processes that include but also exist apart from individual people's experiences.

Occupational science has thus challenged occupational therapy's long-standing conceptualization of occupation as an individualized, intrinsically motivated process through which people act on the environment. By moving away from systems-based theories and drawing more heavily on philosophical understandings of human beings, occupational scientists have endeavored to move individual people from the center of inquiries to permit exploration of other important dimensions of occupation, such as its social (Humphry, 2005), political (Pollard, Kronenberg, & Sakellariou, 2008), and collective (Ramugondo & Kronenberg, 2015) nature. Explorations of these other occupational dimensions have, in turn, influenced ideas about adaptation, to which we now shift our attention.

Adaptation

As previously stated, the notions of occupation and adaptation emerged somewhat hand-in-hand in Adolf Meyer's (1922/1977) paper on the philosophy of occupational therapy. Meyer's work inadvertently exerted a strong influence on our founders—and, indeed, our profession and discipline—when he linked engagement in occupation with a person's ability to adapt to daily life problems (Wood, 1995, 1996). Deeper conceptual explorations of adaptation in the 1970s framed *adaptive responses* as "actively created by the person" and emphasized that "adaptation, as an inherently internal process, cannot be externally imposed" (Wood, 1996, p. 628). Those early conceptualizations also described a process whereby adaptive responses were "called forth through interaction with the environment" (Wood, 1996, p. 629). Hence, much of the occupational therapy literature on adaptation emanated from the same person-centric understandings that initially shaped ideas about occupation. Frank's (1996) later definition of adaptation as "a process of selecting and organizing activities (or occupations) to improve life opportunities and enhance quality of life according to the experience of individuals or groups in an ever-changing environment" (p. 50) reinforced such understandings in the early days of occupational science.

Two occupational therapy scholars were primarily responsible for drawing the concepts of occupation and adaptation together in an explicit way. Schkade and Schultz (1992) attributed "equal importance to the occupational environment, the person, and their interaction" (p. 830) in conceiving the notion of *occupational adaptation*. In defining occupational adaptation, Schkade and Schultz assumed that "occupation provides the means by which human beings adapt to changing needs and conditions" (p. 829) and that mastery is the individual goal that drives adaptive processes. These assumptions echoed and elaborated on the ideas that Adolf Meyer asserted in his seminal paper. At the time of its inception, Schkade and Schultz's Occupational Adaptation framework was consistent with the profession and discipline's shared focus on occupation as an individual experience and their use of systems theories to explain human behavior. Most of the subsequent conceptual development related to occupational adaptation has been located within occupational therapy rather than occupational science, and applications of the concept have reinforced the understanding of occupational adaptation "as primarily an individual's response to intrinsic and extrinsic factors" (Bontje, Kinébanian, Josephsson, & Tamura, 2004, p. 140; Johnson, 2006; Kielhofner, 2008). Although the proposed goal of adaptive processes has shifted in recent conceptualizations from mastery (George, Schkade, & Ishee, 2004) to competence, identity, and the satisfaction of needs and desires (Kielhofner, 2008; Law et al., 1996), occupational adaptation has retained its framing as primarily an individual and intrinsic phenomenon.

Occupational scientists have dedicated less attention to developing the concept of adaptation than the concept of occupation, but their thinking about both concepts has taken similar paths. As noted previously, Malcolm Cutchin (2004) critiqued the profession's understanding of the environment, and he applied this critique directly to the notion of adaptation. Cutchin's critique rested on three points: (1) that the traditional notion of adaptation incorrectly characterized people as existing in relationship to an environmental container (as opposed to living through connected environments); (2) that the motivation for adaptation was always explained as coming from inside an individual (as opposed to the interplay of person and environment); and (3) that the process of adaptation was represented too mechanically due to an overreliance on linear, systems-based theoretical perspectives. Predating the introduction of the transactional perspective, Cutchin (2004) offered the Deweyan notion of *place integration* as an alternate concept to adaptation. He defined place integration as a "process of action to address the problematic aspect of the situation, and thereby remake the situation and bring harmony to our ongoing transactions with it" (p. 309). Problematic situations are ones in which habits cease to support actions that allow people to function; such situations prompt us to become consciously aware of our need to (re)integrate with (not adapt to) place and reconstruct our situations. In contrast to traditional understandings of adaptation, in which environments call forth adaptive responses, Cutchin's notion of place integration highlighted the ways in which the person-environment relationship is always evolving given the continuity of experience and time. In addition, it foregrounded the social and historical values that shape individual experiences of and responses to problematic situations, thus helping broaden the conceptual focus beyond individuals' intrinsic motivations.

The ways in which occupational scientists have taken up place integration illustrate a continued commitment to challenging linear and individually focused conceptions of action. For example, Johansson, Cutchin, & Lilja (2012) used place integration to explain the ways in which older adults' home modification processes were driven by multiple influences in the person-place whole, including the expectations of older adults, health care providers, and larger governmental structures that provided funds for home modifications. Likewise, Heatwole Shank and Cutchin (2010) identified processes of coordinated change and meaning for older women who were living at home despite challenges of older age. Those women's occupations were closely shaped by the home and neighborhood context: Their occupations of doing daily errands with a walker, socializing with neighbors, or quilting had been adjusted, readjusted, and evolved over time as the person-place relationship changed. The place-integrating processes that Heatwole Shank and Cutchin investigated were ongoing, never complete, and oriented toward future meaningful participation instead of being a response to challenging circumstances. Other scholars have continued to develop the concept of occupational adaptation with a broader focus on the social dimensions that Cutchin (2004) and others have highlighted. For instance, Nayar and Stanley's (2015) study on immigration and aging underscored that occupational adaptation is not solely an internal, individual process but rather a social one that can occur both in everyday life and following changes in life circumstances. Nayar and Stanley defined occupational adaptation as "a process that occurs over time and ultimately involves a conscious choice in new ways of doing that are, to some degree, influenced by social relationships and the interactions people have with their environments" (p. 35).

The development of ideas about place integration and occupational adaptation in occupational science augments the discipline's movement beyond individualistic and internally focused conceptualizations of human action. The application of Deweyan philosophical ideas across the notions of occupation and adaptation underscores the ongoing, never-complete nature of action and the ways in which it is always situated through person-environment relationships. In the next section, we will connect these developments with the concept of participation, which has historically been construed as the outcome of successful occupational adaptation.

Participation

In 2001, when the World Health Organization (WHO) published a revised version of the *International Classification of Functioning, Disability and Health* (ICF), the term *participation* became inextricably linked to concepts of health and well-being in the discourses of many health-promoting and rehabilitative disciplines, including occupational therapy (Hemmingsson & Jonsson, 2005). Indeed, the central location of *activity* in the ICF model (WHO, 2001, p. 18) reinforced the basic paradigm of occupational therapy: activity (occupation) and participation contribute directly to individual health. Use of the term *participation* has since proliferated in occupational therapy literature, due in part to the congruence between the WHO (2001) definition of participation as "involvement in a life situation" (p. 213) and existing understandings of occupation "as a type of activity which involves some sort of participation by the individual" (Gray, 1997, p. 9). Simply put, participation was integrated into our lexicon as a synonym for the *doing* of occupation. Consistent with the prevailing understanding of occupation as individualized and intrinsically motivated, participation became enshrined in client-centered practice texts as an enabling principle by which autonomous agents could be "involved in action to help themselves" (Townsend & Landry, 2005, p. 505).

In research on occupation up to the present time, participation has been primarily conceptualized as an individualized and subjective *performance* of an occupation. For example, occupational therapists have researched and described the participation of older adults' experiences of "everyday doings" (Larsson, Haglund, & Hagberg, 2009), of individuals with physical disabilities (Nicklasson & Jonsson, 2012), and of people with chronic pain (Borell, Asaba, Rosenberg, Schult, & Townsend, 2006) or mental illness (Blank, Harries, & Reynolds, 2015). These studies draw on first-person accounts (such as interviews) and use narrative and phenomenological analyses to understand the individual experience of participation, mirroring individualistic ways of characterizing occupation as an internal, individualized, and subjective experience. Another feature of this body of literature is that participation has generally been assumed to have a positive influence—as depicted in the ICF (WHO, 2001)—on an individual's health. For example, participation is positively represented as contributing to mental illness recovery (Blank et al., 2015) or seen as an indicator that barriers have been removed and an individual is enabled to engage as they wish (Sharp, Dunford, & Seddon, 2012).

In recent years, there have been significant critiques of both the WHO ICF and the term *participation* more specifically. For example, Hemmingsson and Jonsson (2005) highlighted limitations of the ICF's ability to address the complexity and interrelationships of multiple occupations that occur simultaneously. Hammell (2015) extended this line of critique in her analysis of the framework's limitations in dealing with "structural and environmental barriers" (p. 81) to participation, as well as the problematic exclusion of subjective meaning and many social and relational dimensions of participation. As the discipline of occupational science has grown and matured, many scholars have also pointed to the limitations in how participation has been conceptualized. Three key contributions from occupational scientists about the phenomenon of participation that challenge and expand our discourse include (1) acknowledging the socially situated nature of participation, (2) articulating dimensions of participation beyond *doing*, and (3) describing the complexity of meaning—at different levels—associated with participation.

Since the early 2000s, there has been a widespread push to acknowledge and describe the social nature of participation, including the cultural influences that shape how and when an occupation is done, as well as how it might change over time (Hocking, Wright-St. Clair, & Bunrayong, 2002). Recent occupational science research has foregrounded how the social environment acts to support or constrain occupation (Hart & Heatwole Shank, 2016; Jones, Hocking, & McPherson, 2016; Laliberte Rudman, Huot, & Dennhardt, 2009); how occupational identity does not emerge from within an individual but is both constructed and changed through participation in a social group (Vrkljan & Polgar, 2007) and is subject to renegotiation within a societal frame of reference (Soeker, 2011); and how occupation can arise collectively among a group of individuals who are jointly participating in shared contexts such as a playground (Jones et al., 2016) or a family home in a Greek town (Kantarzis & Molineux, 2014). Participation in society has also been described in the context of sociopolitical tensions (Sakiyama, Josephsson, & Asaba, 2010), as well as the tensions that often exist in public places in the built and structured environments where participation occurs (Hart & Heatwole Shank, 2016). Instead of treating participation as an individually experienced action, these authors are aligned with a transactional perspective of occupation that situates participation in a particular social context and views occupations as unfolding in socially and historically mediated ways.

Occupational science research has also identified dimensions of participation beyond simply the performance or *doing* of an occupation. If occupational adaptation is "a process rather than a state" (Nayar & Stanley, 2015, p. 27), it follows that participation can be part of that unfolding process over time, linking the past with the imagined future (Vrkljan & Polgar, 2007). From this perspective, adaptation becomes part of the "relational action" that Cutchin et al. (2008) described: adaptation does not *lead* to occupation, but rather *occurs through* participation in occupation. This relational perspective has opened the door for novel inquiries. For example, Jones et al. (2016) studied shared occupations of children with traumatic brain injuries and identified participation-enabling "skills" that were practiced by the children to mutually support and extend their collective participation. Similarly, Heatwole Shank and Cutchin (2016) found that if participation in occupation shapes and is shaped by social values and norms, then individuals' imagination and communication about and arrangement and prioritization of occupations serves to challenge or perpetuate tacit values. Other scholars have argued that participation in an occupation is possible through observing others via a virtual medium such as online messaging or games (Kennedy & Lynch, 2016); via belonging to or identifying with a group such as a service organization, even when not directly performing the service (Heatwole Shank, 2018); or by *cognitive reframing*, whereby an individual may mentally participate in imagining, remembering, or projecting his or her own action in a situation when he or she is not physically or socially present (Heatwole Shank & Cutchin, 2010). These ideas that individuals can participate even when geographically or temporally separate from the performance of a particular occupation make understandings of the ways humans take part in daily life more inclusive.

Finally, scholars have critically examined the tacit assumption that participation leads to positive well-being and meaning. Just as Meyer (1922/1977) influenced the linkage of occupation and adaptation, other early writers and leaders in occupational therapy (Reilly, 1962) influenced the profession's assumption that occupations are linked to increased health and well-being. As occupational scientists have sought to understand occupation itself (Hocking, 2009), the range of meanings associated with participating in occupation has grown. Potentially negative or health-damaging meanings have been identified. For example, McDougall, Buchanan, and Peterson (2013) described challenges faced by caregivers and their depleted opportunities and resources for adaptation; others have explored participation in potentially harmful or dangerous occupations such as binge drinking (Jennings & Cronin-Davis, 2016) and tagging/graffiti (Russell, 2008). These negative implications can also be less direct: Groups of individuals may be limited in the type or extent of participation in which they engage because of social discourses about what is or is not desirable behavior (Heatwole Shank & Cutchin, 2016). If participation in occupation has multiple types of meaning, then adaptation should also be thought of as having both positive and potentially negative dimensions because it occurs through participation processes that are always in process and uncertain.

Recent occupational science scholarship clarifies the situated and mutually influencing relationship of participation and occupational adaptation. Rather than being an individual output of a successfully adaptive human system, participation is understood by these scholars to be something that is socially shaped, can take multiple forms, and occurs through diverse media and locations. Like occupation and adaptation, participation can also have a "dark side" (Twinley, 2013) that warrants recognition and further exploration in the name of fully understanding human experiences.

Implications

The familiar concepts of occupation, adaptation, and participation have been stretched and reshaped during the first three decades of occupational science inquiry. Many occupational scientists now explore dimensions of occupation beyond its individual meaning and experience, and they also see occupational adaptation as an ongoing process where action arises from situations instead of individuals. Likewise, many occupational scientists see participation as a multidimensional process through which adaptive changes emerge. These more relational and situated understandings of occupation, adaptation, and participation have implications for scholarship and practice beyond the examples outlined previously.

First, if occupation is understood as a manifestation of person-environment relationships, then it is possible to reconsider how adaptation occurs to better support change in problematic situations. Based on the occupational science understandings reviewed previously, adaptations can be seen as occurring within the person-environment relationship where both individual and social factors play a role in shaping possible solutions to a problematic situation. Rather than being viewed as something *applied to* either a person or an environmental element, adaptation is instead better understood as a change in the person-environment relationship that aims to enhance functional coordination and ongoing participation in occupation. Because the person-environment relationship is always changing and never complete (Aldrich & Cutchin, 2013), adaptation cannot be an intervention outcome nor a static change that results in a human system's homeostasis. Instead, adaptations are both planned and provisional, and changes enacted through occupations are oriented toward future possibilities for occupational engagement, role fulfillment, or identity development. These understandings broaden not only the types of phenomena scholars aim to investigate but also practitioners' framings of their efforts with clients. By more clearly understanding the social, relational, and situated natures of occupation, adaptation, and participation, scholars and practitioners alike have a more holistic basis for engaging with complex human subjects. Equipped with this expanded foundation, they may uncover new elements outside personal or physical environmental factors that provide possibilities for altering problematic situations. Such understandings can, in turn, challenge assumptions and generate new therapeutic applications of occupation.

Second, recognizing that occupation, adaptation, and participation are shaped by influences beyond an individual's immediate context lays groundwork for more inclusive and justice-focused practice. The call for occupational therapists to focus on population-level issues began in the late 1990s with the publication of the first edition of *An Occupational Perspective of Health* (Wilcock & Hocking, 2015); now in its third edition, this tome is part of a growing body of literature (see Durocher, Gibson, & Rappolt, 2014) that emphasizes non–individual-level influences on occupational participation and the need for a focus on inclusionary (Whiteford & Hocking, 2012) scholarship and practice. Focusing on non-individual influences on occupational adaptation can raise awareness of populations and issues that may have remained outside the purview of traditional occupational therapy practice (Aldrich, Laliberte Rudman, & Dickie, 2017). Many non-individual influences have been elaborated relative to the notion of occupational injustice, or the idea that factors outside individual control can prevent or hinder people's participation in occupations (Durocher et al., 2014; Stadnyk, Townsend, & Wilcock, 2010). In recent years, newer occupational science constructs have been developed to foreground the socially situated nature of occupational choice (Galvaan, 2015), the systems and structures that shape possibilities for occupational engagement (Laliberte Rudman, 2010), and the ways in which people can liberate themselves from oppressive conditions through occupational consciousness (Ramugondo, 2015). Given the global mandate for occupational therapists to address occupational injustices (Hocking & Townsend, 2015; Sakellariou & Pollard, 2013), scholars are beginning to explore the ways in which occupational therapists can enable occupational justice (Bailliard & Aldrich, 2016; Townsend & Marval, 2013) by drawing on the Occupation-Based Community Development Framework (OBCD; Galvaan & Peters, 2016) or the Participatory Occupational Justice Framework (POJF; Whiteford, Townsend, Bryanton, Wicks, & Pereira, 2016) to guide their practices. Each of these frameworks outlines phases of action (from *initiation* through *monitoring, reflection,* and *evaluation* in the case of OBCD) or enablement skills (from *raising consciousness* through *advocacy and sustainability* in the case of POJF) that can be enacted to build partnerships with communities that feel the effects of occupational injustices. As these explorations move forward, it will be important to see how current understandings of occupational adaptation resonate with attempts to redress exclusion and injustice.

ADVANCING THE KNOWLEDGE ON OCCUPATIONAL ADAPTATION

The therapeutic application of occupation has historically been oriented toward helping individuals overcome challenges of mind and body in order to maximize function. The desired end of occupational therapy practice has long been defined as an agentic individual acting on an external environment, but the advent of occupational science has helped scholars approach core constructs with fresh, critical eyes. Through this critical development, occupational adaption has come to reflect a more nuanced understanding of person-and-environment relationships as co-creating and continuous, with action arising from problematic situations that are contingent, uncertain, and part of a process that is never complete. Through adaptive processes, humans are seen as grappling with and finding meaning in challenging circumstances, not to achieve homeostasis through adaptation but to devise and integrate functional solutions. From this theoretically grounded perspective, occupational therapists and occupational scientists' knowledge about human action and occupational adaptation can be applied to diverse settings and to social, structural, and global issues affecting participation. The final chapter of this book will provide examples of these applications, synthesized from accounts of lived experiences.

Summary and Implications

- The development of occupational science led to a reexamination and expansion of core concepts including occupation, adaptation, and participation.
- Emerging understandings suggest that occupation represents a relationship of person and place, influenced by social and structural dimensions, and not just an individually experienced phenomenon.
- Adaptation is not an action *on* the environment, but a continuous process of action arising from a problematic situation that is oriented toward possible (but never certain) solutions and reintegrations.
- Participation in occupation is the active process through which adaptation occurs and is more complex than the *performance* of an occupation.
- Expanded conceptualizations of occupation, adaptation, and participation have widened the scope of research and therapeutic practice.

References

Aldrich, R. M. (2008). From complexity theory to transactionalism: Moving occupational science forward in theorizing the complexities of behavior. *Journal of Occupational Science, 15*(3), 147-156.

Aldrich, R. M. & Cutchin, M. P. (2013). Dewey's concepts of embodiment, growth and occupation: Extended bases for a transactional perspective. In M. Cutchin & V. Dickie (Eds.), *Transactional perspectives on occupation* (pp. 13-24). Dordrecht, Netherlands: Springer.

Aldrich, R. M., Laliberte Rudman, D., & Dickie, V. A. (2017). Resource seeking as occupation: A critical and empirical exploration. *American Journal of Occupational Therapy, 71*, 7103260010p1-7103260010p9.

Bailliard, A. & Aldrich, R. M. (2016). Occupational justice in everyday occupational therapy practice. In D. Sakellariou & N. Pollard (Eds.), *Occupational therapies without borders: Integrating justice with practice* (pp. 83-94). Edinburgh, Scotland: Elsevier.

Blank., A. A., Harries, P., & Reynolds, F. (2015). 'Without occupation you don't exist': Occupational engagement and mental illness. *Journal of Occupational Science, 22*(2), 197-209.

Bontje, P., Kinébanian, A., Josephsson, S., & Tamura, Y. (2004). Occupational adaptation: The experiences of older persons with physical disabilities. *American Journal of Occupational Therapy, 58*(2), 140-149.

Borell, L., Asaba, E., Rosenberg, L., Schult, M. L., & Townsend, E. (2006). Exploring experiences of "participation" among individuals living with chronic pain. *Scandinavian Journal of Occupational Therapy, 13*, 76-85.

Byrne, D. S. (1998). *Complexity theory and the social sciences: An introduction.* Florence, KY: Routledge.

Christiansen, C. (1994). Classification and study in occupation: A review and discussion of taxonomies. *Journal of Occupational Science, 1*(3), 3-21.

Christiansen, C., Clark, F., Kielhofner, G., Rogers, J., & Nelson, D. (1995). Position paper: Occupation. *American Journal of Occupational Therapy, 49*(10), 1015-1018.

Clark, F. A., Parham, D., Carlson, M. E., Frank, G., Jackson, J., Pierce, D., ... Zemke, R. (1991). Occupational science: Academic innovation in the service of occupational therapy's future. *American Journal of Occupational Therapy, 45*(4), 300-310.

Cutchin, M. P. (2004). Using Deweyan philosophy to rename and reframe adaptation-to-environment. *American Journal of Occupational Therapy, 58*, 303-312.

Cutchin, M. P., Aldrich, R. M., Bailliard, A. L., & Coppola, S. (2008). Action theories for occupational science: The contributions of Dewey and Bourdieu. *Journal of Occupational Science, 15*(3), 157-165.

Cutchin, M. P., & Dickie, V. A. (2013). *Transactional perspectives on occupation.* Dordrecht, Netherlands: Springer.

Dickie, V. A. (2003). The role of learning in quilt making. *Journal of Occupational Science, 10*(3), 120-129.

Dickie, V. A. (2010). Are occupations 'processes too complicated to explain'? What we can learn by trying. *Journal of Occupational Science, 17*(4), 195-203.

Dickie, V. A., Cutchin, M. P., & Humphry, R. (2006). Occupation as transactional experience: A critique of individualism in occupational science. *Journal of Occupational Science, 13*(1), 83-93.

Durocher, E., Gibson, B. E., & Rappolt, S. (2014). Occupational justice: A conceptual review. *Journal of Occupational Science, 21*(4), 418-430. doi:10.1080/14427591.2013.775692

Eakman, A. (2007). Occupation and social complexity. *Journal of Occupational Science, 14*(2), 82-91.

Evans, K. A. (1987). Definition of occupation as the core concept of occupational therapy. *American Journal of Occupational Therapy, 41*(10), 627-628. doi:10.5014/ajot.41.10.627

Frank, G. (1996). The concept of adaptation as a foundation for occupational science research. In R. Zemke & F. Clark (Eds.), *Occupational science: The evolving discipline* (pp. 47-55). Philadelphia, PA: F.A. Davis.

Frank, G. (2012). Occupational therapy/occupational science/occupational justice: Moral commitments and global assemblages. *Journal of Occupational Science, 19*(1), 25-35.

Galvaan, R. (2015). The contextually situated nature of occupational choice: Marginalized young adolescents' experiences in South Africa. *Journal of Occupational Science, 22*(1), 39-53.

Galvaan, R., & Peters, L. (2016). Occupation-based community development: Confronting the politics of occupation. In D. Sakellariou & N. Pollard (Eds.), *Occupational therapies without borders: Integrating justice with practice* (pp. 283-291). Edinburgh, Scotland: Elsevier.

George, L. A., Schkade, J. K., & Ishee, J. H. (2004). Content validity of the Relative Mastery Measurement Scale: A measure of occupational adaptation. *OTJR: Occupation, Participation, and Health, 24*(3), 92-102.

Golledge, J. (1998). Distinguishing between occupation, purposeful activity and activity, part 1: Review and explanation. *British Journal of Occupational Therapy, 61*(3), 100-104.

Gray, J. M. (1997). Application of the phenomenological method to the concept of occupation. *Journal of Occupational Science, 4*(1), 5-17.

Gray, J. M., Kennedy, B. L., & Zemke, R. (1996a). Application of dynamic systems theory to occupation. In R. Zemke & F. Clark (Eds.), *Occupational science: The evolving discipline* (pp. 309-324). Philadelphia, PA: F.A. Davis.

Gray, J. M., Kennedy, B. L., & Zemke, R. (1996b). Dynamic Systems Theory: An overview. In R. Zemke & F. Clark (Eds.), *Occupational science: The evolving discipline* (pp. 297-308). Philadelphia, PA: F.A. Davis.

Hammell, K. W. (2015). Quality of life, participation and occupational rights: A capabilities perspective. *Australian Occupational Therapy Journal, 62*, 78-85. doi:10/1111/1440-1630.12183

Hart, E. C., & Heatwole Shank, K. (2016). Participating at the mall: Possibilities and tensions that shape older adults' occupations. *Journal of Occupational Science,* 1-15. doi:10.1080/14427591.2015.1020851

Heatwole Shank, K. (2018). *Layered purposes of participation.* Manuscript in preparation.

Heatwole Shank, K., & Cutchin, M. P. (2010). Transactional occupations of older women aging-in-place: Negotiating change and meaning. *Journal of Occupational Science, 17*(1), 4-13. doi:10.1080/1442759 1.2010.9686666

Heatwole Shank, K., & Cutchin, M. P. (2016). Processes of negotiating 'community livability' in older age. *Journal of Aging Studies, 39*, 66-72. doi:10.1016/j.jaging.2016.11.001

Hemmingsson, H., & Jonsson, H. (2005). An occupational perspective on the concept of participation in the International classification of function, disability and health—some critical remarks. *American Journal of Occupational Therapy, 59*(5), 569-576.

Henderson, A. (1996). The scope of occupational science. In R. Zemke & F. Clark (Eds.), *Occupational science: The evolving discipline* (pp. 419-424). Philadelphia, PA: F.A. Davis.

Hinojosa, J., Kramer, P., Royeen, C. B., & Luebben, A. J. (2003). Core concept of occupation. In P. Kramer, J. Hinojosa, & C. B. Royeen (Eds.), *Perspectives in human occupation: Participation in life* (pp. 1-17). Philadelphia, PA: Lippincott Williams & Wilkins.

Hocking, C. (2009). The challenge of occupation: Describing the things people do. *Journal of Occupational Science, 16*(3), 140-150.

Hocking, C., & Townsend, E. (2015). Driving social change: Occupational therapists' contributions to occupational justice. *World Federation of Occupational Therapists Bulletin, 71*(2), 68-71. doi:10.1179/2 056607715Y.0000000002

Hocking, C., Wright-St. Clair, V., & Bunrayong, W. (2002). The meaning of cooking and recipe work for older Thai and New Zealand women. *Journal of Occupational Science, 9*(3), 117-127. doi:10.1080/144 27591.2002.9686499

Humphry, R. (2005). Model of processes transforming occupations: Exploring societal and social influences. *Journal of Occupational Science, 12*(1), 36-44.

Jennings, H., & Cronin-Davis, J. (2016). Investigating binge drinking using interpretative phenomenological analysis: Occupation for health or harm? *Journal of Occupational Science, 23*(2), 245-254.

Johansson, K., Cutchin, M. P., & Lilja, M. (2012). Place integration: A conceptual tool to understand the home modification process. In M. Cutchin & V.A. Dickie (Eds.), *Transactional perspectives on occupation* (pp. 107-117). Dordrecht, Netherlands: Springer.

Johnson, J. A. (2006). Describing the phenomenon of homelessness through the theory of occupational adaptation. *Occupational Therapy in Health Care, 20*(3/4), 63-80.

Jones, M., Hocking, C., & McPherson, K. (2016). Communities with participation-enabling skills: A study of children with traumatic brain injury and their shared occupations. *Journal of Occupational Science, 24*(1), 88-104. doi:10.1080/14427591.2016.1224444

Kantartzis, S., & Molineux, M. (2014). Occupation to maintain the family as ideology and practice in a Greek town. *Journal of Occupational Science, 21*(3), 277-295. doi:10.1080/14427591.2014.908480

Kennedy, J., & Lynch, H. (2016). A shift from offline to online: Adolescence, the internet and social participation. *Journal of Occupational Science, 23*(2), 156-167. doi:10.1080/14427591.2015.1117523

Kielhofner, G. (2008). *Model of Human Occupation: Theory and application* (4th ed.). Baltimore, MD: Lippincott Williams & Wilkins.

Kielhofner, G., & Burke, J. P. (1977). Occupational therapy after 60 years: An account of changing identity and knowledge. *American Journal of Occupational Therapy, 31*(10), 675-689.

Kielhofner, G., & Burke, J. P. (1980). A model of human occupation, part 1: Conceptual framework and content. *American Journal of Occupational Therapy, 34*(9), 572-581.

Laliberte Rudman, D. (2010). Occupational terminology: Occupational possibilities. *Journal of Occupational Science, 17*(1), 55-59.

Laliberte Rudman, D. (2013). Enacting the critical potential of occupational science: Problematizing the 'individualizing of occupation'. *Journal of Occupational Science, 4*, 298-313. doi:10.1080/14427591.2 013.803434

Laliberte Rudman, D., & Aldrich, R. M. (2017). Occupational science. In M. Curtin, M. Egan, & J. Adams (Eds.), *Occupational therapy for people experiencing illness, injury or impairment: Promoting occupation and participation* (7th ed., pp. 17-27). New York, NY: Elsevier.

Laliberte Rudman, D., Huot, S., & Dennhardt, S. (2009). Shaping ideal places for retirement: Occupational possibilities within contemporary media. *Journal of Occupational Science, 16*(1), 18-24. doi:10.1 080/14427591.2009.9686637

Larsson, A., Haglund, L., & Hagberg, J. (2009). Doing everyday life—experiences of the oldest old. *Scandinavian Journal of Occupational Therapy, 16*(2), 99-109. doi:10.1080/11038120802409762

Law, M., Cooper, B., Strong, S., Stewart, D., Rigby, P., & Letts, L. (1996). The Person-Environment-Occupation Model: A transactive approach to occupational performance. *Canadian Journal of Occupational Therapy, 63*(1), 9-23.

McDougall, C., Buchanan, A., & Peterson, S. (2013). Understanding primary carers' occupational adaptation and engagement. *Australian Occupational Therapy Journal, 61*, 83-91. doi:10.1111/1440-1630.12076

Meyer, A. (1977). The philosophy of occupation therapy. *American Journal of Occupational Therapy, 31*(10), 639-642. (Reprinted from Archives of Occupational Therapy, 1922, 1, pp. 1-10.)

Molineux, M., & Whiteford, G. E. (2011). Occupational science: Genesis, evolution and future contribution. In E. A. S. Duncan (Ed.), *Foundations for practice in occupational therapy* (pp. 243-253).

Molke, D. K., Laliberte Rudman, D., & Polatajko, H. J. (2004). The promise of occupational science: A developmental assessment of an emerging academic discipline. *Canadian Journal of Occupational Therapy, 71*(5), 269-280.

Nayar, S., & Stanley, M. (2015). Occupational adaptation as a social process in everyday life. *Journal of Occupational Science, 22*(1), 26-38.

Nicklasson, M., & Jonsson, H. (2012). Experience of participation as described by people with hand deformity cause by rheumatic disease. *British Journal of Occupational Therapy, 75*, 29-35.

Occupational terminology interactive dialogue. (2001). *Journal of Occupational Science, 8*(2), 38-41.

Pierce, D. (2001). Untangling occupation and activity. *American Journal of Occupational Therapy, 55*(2), 138-146.

Pierce, D. (2012). The 2011 Ruth Zemke lecture in occupational science: Promise. *Journal of Occupational Science, 19*(4), 298-311.

Pollard, N., Kronenberg, F., & Sakellariou, D. (2008). A political practice of occupational therapy. In N. Pollard, D. Sakellariou, & F. Kronenberg (Eds.), *A political practice of occupational therapy* (pp. 3-19). Edinburgh, Scotland: Churchill Livingstone.

Ramugondo, E. (2015). Occupational terminology: Occupational consciousness. *Journal of Occupational Science, 22*(4), 488-501.

Ramugondo, E., & Kronenberg, F. (2015). Explaining collective occupations from a human relations perspective: Bridging the individual-collective dichotomy. *Journal of Occupational Science, 22*(1), 3-16.

Reilly, M. (1962). The Eleanor Clarke Slagle: Occupational therapy can be one of the great ideas of 20th century medicine. *American Journal of Occupational Therapy, 16*(1), 1-9.

Royeen, C. B. (2002). Occupation reconsidered. *Occupational Therapy International, 9*(2), 111-120.

Russell, E. (2008). The writing on the wall: The form, function, and meaning of tagging. *Journal of Occupational Science, 15*(2), 87-97.

Sakellariou, D., & Pollard, N. (2013). A commentary on the social responsibility of occupational therapy education. *Journal of Further and Higher Education, 37*(3), 416-430. doi:10.1080/030987 7X.2011.645459

Sakiyama, M., Josephsson, S., & Asaba, E. (2010). What is participation? A story of mental illness, metaphor, & everyday occupation. *Journal of Occupational Science, 17*(4), 224-230. doi:10.1080/1442759 1.2010.9686699

Schkade, J. K., & Schultz, S. (1992). Occupational adaptation: Toward a holistic approach for contemporary practice, part 1. *American Journal of Occupational Therapy, 46*(9), 829-837.

Schwartz, K. B. (2003). History of occupation. In P. Kramer, J. Hinojosa, & C. B. Royeen (Eds.), *Perspectives in human occupation: Participation in life* (pp. 18-31). Philadelphia, PA: Lippincott Williams & Wilkins.

Sharp, N., Dunford, C., & Seddon, L. (2012). A critical appraisal of how occupational therapists can enable participation in adaptive physical activity for children and young people. *British Journal of Occupational Therapy, 75*(11), 486-494. doi:10.4276/030802212X13522194759815

Soeker, M. S. (2011). Occupational adaptation: A return to work perspective of persons with mild to moderate brain injury in South Africa. *Journal of Occupational Science, 18*(1), 81-91. doi:10.1080/144275 91.2011.554155

Stadnyk, R. L., Townsend, E. A., & Wilcock, A. A. (2010). Occupational justice. In C. Christiansen & E. Townsend (Eds.), *Introduction to occupation: The art and science of living* (2nd ed., pp. 329-358). Upper Saddle River, NJ: Pearson.

Townsend, E., & Landry, J. (2005). Interventions in a societal context: Enabling participation. In C. H. Christiansen, C. M. Baum, & J. Bass-Haugen (Eds.), *Occupational therapy: Performance, participation and well-being* (3rd ed., pp. 495-520). Thorofare, NJ: SLACK Incorporated.

Townsend, E., & Marval, R. (2013). Can professionals actually enable occupational justice? *Cadernos de Terapia Ocupacional da UFSCar, 21*(2), 215-228. doi:10.4322/cto.2013.025

Twinley, R. (2013). The dark side of occupation: A concept for consideration. *Australian Occupational Therapy Journal, 60*, 301-303. doi:10.1111/1440-1630.12026

von Bertalanffy, V. L. (1962). *General Systems Theory*. New York, NY: George Braziller.

Vrkljan, B. H., & Polgar, J. M. (2007). Linking occupational participation and occupational identity: An exploratory study of the transition from driving to driving cessation in older adulthood. *Journal of Occupational Science, 14*(1), 30-39.

Whiteford, G. E., & Hocking, C. (2012). *Occupational science: Society, inclusion, participation*. West Sussex, England: Wiley-Blackwell.

Whiteford, G. E., Townsend, E., Bryanton, O., Wicks, A., & Pereira, R. (2016). The Participatory Occupational Justice Framework: Salience across contexts. In D. Sakellariou & N. Pollard (Eds.), *Occupational therapies without borders: Integrating justice with practice* (pp. 163-174). Edinburgh, Scotland: Elsevier.

Whiteford, G. E., Townsend, E., & Hocking, C. (2000). Reflections on a renaissance of occupation. *Canadian Journal of Occupational Therapy, 67*(1), 61-69.

Wilcock, A. A., & Hocking, C. (2015). *An occupational perspective of health* (3rd ed.). Thorofare, NJ: SLACK Incorporated.

Wood, W. (1995). Weaving the warp and weft of occupational therapy: An art and science for all times. *American Journal of Occupational Therapy, 49*(1), 44-52.

Wood, W. (1996). Legitimizing occupational therapy's knowledge. *American Journal of Occupational Therapy, 58*(8), 626-634.

World Health Organization. (2001). *International classification of function, disability and health*. Geneva, Switzerland: Author.

Wright-St. Clair, V., Hocking, C., Bunrayong, W., Vittayakorn, S., & Rattakorn, P. (2005). Older New Zealand women doing the work of Christmas: A recipe for identity formation. *Sociological Review, 53*(2), 332-350.

Wu, C., & Lin, K. (1999). Defining occupation: A comparative analysis. *Journal of Occupational Science, 6*(1), 5-12.

Yerxa, E. J., Clark, F., Jackson, J., Pierce, D., & Zemke, R. (1990). An introduction to occupational science: A foundation for occupational therapy in the 21st century. *Occupational Therapy in Health Care, 6*(4), 1-17.

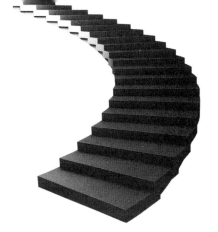

10

The Lived Experience of Occupational Adaptation

Adaptation in the Wake of Adversity, Life Transitions, and Change

Mandy Stanley, PhD

OVERVIEW In this chapter, *occupational adaptation* is defined as the process that unfolds when a person is faced with occupational disruption or an occupational challenge. The individual engages in the occupational adaptation process with the intention to achieve mastery over the occupations that were challenging or make a decision to replace occupations that previously held value and meaning to the person. Several themes will be presented to broaden the applications of occupational adaptation in humans as occupational beings as evidenced by several research studies on the lived experiences of clients. During major life transitions, occupational adaptation is a process of:

- Engaging in new occupations and accepting new ways of doing
- Navigating new occupational roles and adjusting value systems
- Building a new sense of self-belief
- A transaction with familiar and new environments
- Reconfiguring identity, choices, and sense of control

Grajo LC, Boisselle AK, eds.
Adaptation Through Occupation:
Multidimensional Perspectives (pp 175-192).
© 2019 SLACK Incorporated.

CHAPTER OBJECTIVES By the end of this chapter, the reader will be able to:
- Describe ways of studying the experience or process of occupational adaptation.
- Identify common elements of occupational adaptation across the studies.
- Identify gaps in knowledge about the experience of occupational adaptation.

QUESTIONS FOR DISCUSSION AND REFLECTION As the reader explores this chapter, let the following questions guide discussion and reflection:
- How does restructuring identity and finding new or reclaimed occupation play a role in the adaptation process following disability or difficult life transitions?
- In what ways do choice and control in occupational engagement influence occupational adaptation?

INTRODUCTION

To begin the chapter, I am going to start with two stories about transition. These stories set the scene, and I will return to the stories later in the chapter to consider them again in light of the knowledge gained from the research about occupational adaptation. They involve fictional characters and are not anyone's story but are based on real situations. Any relationship of these stories to real people is purely accidental but perhaps reflects the common occurrence of the transitions.

Daniel's Story

Daniel is a geologist whose job involves shift work flying in and out of mine and exploration sites at a distance from home for 10 days at a time. He has been recently laid off due to financial slowdowns in the economy and reduction of mining exploration by the big mining companies. This is the second time that Daniel has been retrenched in the past 20 years. Daniel is 53 years old and has a partner and two adult children.

Beulah's Story

Beulah was married for 48 years until her husband Silas died recently. Silas had Alzheimer's disease, and Beulah cared for him at home until his death. Beulah's day revolved around looking after Silas' personal care needs as well as managing all the household tasks with support from family members. Her health is quite good, although she does have a little arthritis. Beulah misses Silas but is grateful that he no longer suffers the indignity of not being able to look after himself.

Having set the scene with the stories of Daniel and Beulah, we come to recognize that there are many transitions in life that occur across the life span. Some are planned, wanted, and anticipated, such as starting school, leaving home, becoming a parent, and retiring from paid employment. Other transitions are sudden and catastrophic, such as a major illness, the death of a family member, a natural disaster, or loss of employment. All of these transitions have an impact on occupational engagement and require occupational adaptation. We will return to the stories later in the chapter.

In this chapter, the focus is on the lived experience of occupational adaptation. I will draw on a number of research studies that I have been involved with to inform my discussion along with some of the published literature. I will then draw together the common threads across the discussion in an attempt to reveal what is known about occupational adaptation and how these studies develop the understandings.

Occupational Adaptation Following Brain Injury, Stroke, and End-Stage Renal Disease

The first study that I draw on is a small qualitative study of two young men, Gus and Eric (pseudonyms), following brain injury who were living in rural areas (Parsons & Stanley, 2008). We were interested in finding out about their experience of occupational adaptation following their return to living in their rural community. It is known that young men coming from rural areas have a higher incidence of brain injury (Hillier, Hillier, & Metzer, 1997) due to the greater propensity for engagement in risk-taking behaviors. The incidence has reduced in recent years due to the introduction of road safety policies (Beck, Bray, Cameron, Cooper, & Gabbe, 2016), yet people living with brain injury in rural areas have less access to rehabilitation services than their urban counterparts, and little was known about how they might adapt. Both Gus' and Eric's lives changed drastically as the young men went from having busy, active lives working and socializing to lives impacted by complex and multiple impairments.

Immediately following the injury and for some time afterward, the young men had difficulty coming to terms with their changed bodies and altered capacities. In time, they had to accept that things were different now to learn new ways of doing. They had to change the manner in which they lived in order to move forward into another chapter in their lives. *Engaging in new occupations* enabled them to learn the importance of those new occupations as being meaningful and relevant as well as enjoyable. The familiar support systems of family, friends, and the rural community played a large part in occupational adaptation. Although access to specialist brain injury support services may have been lacking in the rural communities in which Gus and Eric lived, they did have the advantage of the community acceptance and support, which may not be the case in urban or city area.

The findings from this small study are supported by another small qualitative study of occupational adaptation of persons with mild to moderate brain injury on returning to work in the Western Cape in South Africa (Soeker, 2011). The 10 participants described a similar loss of the former self, both in terms of loss of capacities and loss of future aspirations and occupational roles, and in terms of facing an uncertain future. Participants *built a new sense of self-belief* and acceptance with support from family. Participation in occupation enabled growth and recovery in changing the way that they did things to match the new reduced capacities but also to provide a structure and routine. For most, the return to work was to a different work role in a different capacity that was a better match with their abilities following brain injury.

In another Australian study, this time following stroke or acquired brain injury rather than traumatic brain injury, Williams and Murray (2013) interviewed three men and two women who ranged from 1.5 to 14 years post-stroke. Immediately post-stroke, the participants had experienced a period of shock because their whole lives had changed and they were no longer the people they thought they were. Once the shock began to wear off, they realized that they had to get on and do their best and to learn to adjust to the new life. From shock, they moved to a willingness to overcome problems and try new things. Participants spoke of stretching the limitations to find out what they could and couldn't do but also to extend the limitations further. They held on to hope that they would improve, but, in the meantime, they had to *accept new ways of doing*.

This is in contrast to people who were recovering from stroke is a study of Mexican Americans in end-stage renal disease (Wells, 2015). The 17 participants had been on dialysis from 6 to 132 months and experienced a heightened awareness of their mortality. The routine of dialysis provided a structure to the week that kept reminding the person and the family of how unwell the person was and the lack of control that they had over the illness. In addition, the dialysis robbed them of the freedom to engage in usual occupations, including work, because of the need to spend 3 to 4 hours, three times a week on dialysis. The condition impacted social occupations because they could not drink alcohol, and they withdrew from social situations in which they would have to explain to others about their condition. Having a fistula meant that swimming or taking a bath were occupations that had to be avoided and impacted what the person chose to wear. Travel was another freedom that was lost. Participants had to accept the restrictions of freedom and impact on occupational engagement in order to remain alive and well.

OCCUPATIONAL ADAPTATION IN PARENTING AND CAREGIVING OF PRE-TERM INFANTS

From transitioning back to the community following head injury or stroke and living with end-stage renal disease, I turn to a very different transition now: that of becoming a parent to a pre-term infant. We conducted a meta-ethnography of 35 studies of experiences of parenting in the neonatal intensive care unit (Gibbs, Boshoff, & Stanley, 2015). A meta-ethnographic synthesis brings together the findings from a number of qualitative studies and, through interpretive analysis, arrives at findings at a higher conceptual level than could be achieved from a single study. When parents had a baby who was pre-term, they were faced with the unanticipated reality of the neonatal intensive care unit. They had to relinquish the ideas that they had around the birth and holding a brand-new baby and then taking the infant home after a few days. They then had to adapt to the strange, unfamiliar technical environment of the neonatal intensive care unit. They also had to relinquish the parenting role and allow the medical and nursing staff to provide care when the infants' health was fragile. Parents were left feeling vulnerable and powerless and juggling roles and responsibilities, such as caring for other children at home or fulfilling work responsibilities. Gradually they began to (re)claim an alternative parental role, becoming more familiar with the environment, coming to know the baby, and developing partnerships with staff. It was through engaging in caregiving occupations that they built confidence and began to adapt to the role of parenting a pre-term infant.

We followed the meta-ethnographic synthesis with a primary study in which three sets of parents were interviewed about their experiences parenting a pre-term infant (Gibbs, Boshoff, & Stanley, 2016). Analysis of the parents' stories revealed a similar process of occupational adaptation to the meta-ethnography. The study revealed ways in which parents worked to reclaim the parental role through participating in occupations that gave them meaning as parents. These occupations included becoming involved in breastfeeding, supplemental bottle or tube feeding, and bathing. However, the ability to perform the parenting occupations was *impacted by the environment*; for example, there were no privacy screens for a mother who was learning to breastfeed her infant. They had to navigate the neonatal intensive care unit *occupation-environment transactions*, including the presence of intensive care equipment, lines, and respiratory equipment, in order to maintain a connection with the baby. The culture of the unit also impacted parenting occupations, with parents being excluded during ward rounds. Staff on the unit acted as gatekeepers to the infants, so parents built relationships with staff to obtain information and the creation of opportunities to participate in parenting occupations. Gradually the parents created a revised version of the anticipated future, which for some included the possibility of their child having ongoing issues due to prematurity. The findings from this study and the meta-ethnography provide guidance for how parents might be able to engage in parenting occupations from an early stage in order to assist the process of occupational adaptation.

I turn now from caring for pre-term infants to caring for someone with an intellectual disability living in a remote rural area in Western Australia (McDougall, Buchanan, & Peterson, 2014). The eight caregivers interviewed in the study were predominantly female and had been caregiving for an average of 25 years. Caregivers *adapted to their role* by prioritizing the care recipient's needs over their own, with the occupations involved in providing care taking precedence over other occupations. Prioritizing caring occupations enabled them to learn new occupations but was a barrier to other occupational engagement, particularly leisure occupations. Performing the lifelong commitment of the caregiver role well meant that they always had to put others first. If caregivers had good quality supports, they were able to relax knowing that the care recipients were being cared for, which enabled engagement in other pleasurable occupations for respite. In the rural context, there was considerable support within the small community. Caregivers' visions for the future involved caregiving occupations becoming harder due to aging and having concerns about future care for the care recipients if the caregivers could no longer perform that role.

GROUNDED THEORY STUDIES ON OCCUPATIONAL ADAPTATION

Much of the academic attention paid to occupational adaptation has been studying people with a disability, which is not surprising given that most occupational therapists work with people with a disability and given the strong connection between occupational therapy and occupational science. Walder and Molineux (2017) conducted a rigorous synthesis of qualitative studies on the experience of adjusting to chronic disease or a significant health event. Following a systematic search, they analyzed 37 studies using a grounded theory analysis (Eaves, 2001) in order to generate a theory about an underlying process of reconstructing an occupational identity. People living with chronic disease or who have experienced a significant health event experience turmoil and loss. They use the processes of *developing competence, finding motivation*, and *becoming confident* in order to achieve occupational adaptation and to *reconstruct their occupational identity*. Each of these processes comprises sub-categories related to mastery and acceptance; adjusting to change; building hope, a sense of belonging, and a feeling of being needed; making a contribution; overcoming fear; and forming routines. The synthesis shows that reconstructing one's identity and finding new purpose and meaning in life are vitally important to occupational adaptation and occupational well-being.

The study of caregivers in the previous section, together with the findings from the synthesis of studies of people living with chronic conditions, show the application to other occupational roles and transitions. Another example comes from the work of Nayar and Stanley (2014) in using grounded theory to explore how Indian immigrant women settle in their adopted country of New Zealand. Using both interviews and observations, data were collected from 25 Indian women and analyzed using constant comparative analysis and drawing on Schatzman's (1991) dimensional analysis. The resultant theory about the process of navigating cultural spaces included a category of shaping self as a strategy to facilitate occupational engagement.

Shaping self involved dimensions of presenting self and hiding self as Indian. The women chose at different times to openly and actively engage with Indian culture and the Indian community in New Zealand or to hide the self as Indian by engaging in ways that fitted with New Zealand and letting ties to India be relinquished. Actively engaging with the Indian community and culture enabled the women to practice certain occupations in a space that was familiar and where they were with people with similar values. There was a sense of feeling safe that came from knowing what to expect. The home was also a place where the women could practice Indian culture in the way they dressed, spoke their own language, cooked Indian food, and went about daily occupations in familiar ways.

Hiding self as Indian was to deny the Indian cultural heritage and to render the identity as an Indian woman invisible. Adopting New Zealand practices facilitated integrating and creating new connections while relinquishing ties to Indian culture and practices. Sometimes the New Zealand practices were not compatible with Indian cultural values, such as dressing in shorts and sleeveless tops or consuming alcohol. Relinquishing ties included not wearing traditional clothing of saris and churidhars but saving them for special occasions and wearing more acceptable clothing for New Zealand, such as trousers and skirts. It also included internal changes, such as changing attitude to fit with attitudes in New Zealand. Shaping self was a strategy used for occupational adaptation within the adopted country.

In my own doctoral work, I conducted a classical grounded theory study of how older people in Australia achieve and maintain well-being (Stanley, 2009). I interviewed 15 older people living in the community in one Australian city to derive a theory of well-being with the core category being *perceived control*, in which the older people utilized a basic social process of *trading off*. As people age, there are changes to capacity and events, such as loss of a partner, ill health, loss of a pet, or some such challenge to equilibrium. The change in capacity of the person may result in a mismatch between the demands of the occupation and the environment, impacting occupational performance. If it was not possible to boost the capacities of the person back to what they were or to modify the environment, then older people used trading off to manage and adapt to the situation. The first phase in trading off was to recognize the issue with occupational performance. In the second phase, older people considered the choices available to them and evaluated the advantages and disadvantages of the options. The third and final phase involved making a choice about which action to take. Generally speaking, there are several different forms of trading off that can be considered and evaluated; they are expanded on here with examples.

Older people can exchange the occupation from one that is no longer within their capacities to one that is, and one that is similar in terms of interests, values, and satisfaction. For example, one of the participants in my doctoral study, Bev, used to enjoy line dancing; however, her back condition prevented her from engaging without pain. She decided to discontinue line dancing but wanted an occupation that still provided her with the ability to exercise in order to keep fit and active as she aged. She chose to take up swimming and found a pool that she could walk to in the morning in the next suburb, which met her need to exercise relatively pain free.

Instead of trading off what occupation is engaged in, it is possible to *trade how the occupation is performed*. For example, a couple I interviewed had always been highly social and gave a lot of dinner parties. Now that Radlee had a high level of incapacity due to Parkinson's disease and Hubert's role involved that of her caregiver, they were not able to engage in that social occupation. Hubert had to take over much of the cooking and dinner party planning, even if it was not part of his culinary repertoire. Also, the couple was too tired at the end of the day to entertain. They now held afternoon tea parties, which were much simpler to prepare and clean up and were at a time of day they could manage. This enabled the couple to be the gracious social hosts they wanted to be. Trading off occupations in this way enabled them to have a sense of perceived control.

Another alternative use of trading off was to give the responsibility for occupational engagement in the troublesome area to someone else. The *allocation of occupations* to someone else is a common response for older people as they age and lose capacities and could easily be viewed as a sign of increasing dependence and concurrent loss of independence. When trading off is used, it is as a conscious decision of the older person who chooses what it is he or she allocates to someone else and who to assign it to. The driver for using trading off is to maintain perceived control and to achieve a higher-order goal such as remaining in one's own living space. Obvious examples of this type of trading off are house cleaning, cooking, and shopping, where the older person chooses to have these tasks performed by a family member or friend or to pay for the service. Exercising trading off in this way is an act of exerting one's agency and self-determination with a small concurrent loss of independence.

The final way that trading off can be exercised is to *change one's values*. The older person needs to accept that the occupation he or she can no longer perform is not important to him or her and can be discarded without a cost to the self apart from an adjustment of the value system. Examples of this form of trading off include accepting wrinkled clothes or clothes that don't need ironing if ironing is difficult to perform, or accepting a lower standard of cleanliness and presentation if house cleaning is too difficult and beyond the person's capacity. Although the older person may be comfortable in accepting the change of values, there may be repercussions with family members or other outsiders who view the older person as not coping when he or she is indeed making occupational adaptations.

The use of trading off in one or more of the ways described is an *adaptive response* to changes in the circumstances of aging. It can be the result of a conscious choice, similar to the choices made by the Indian immigrant women who made choices about how they revealed or showed their Indian ways to meet the demands of the environment. The findings from both of these studies provide examples of occupational adaptation in the everyday and show that occupational adaptation is an ongoing and dynamic process.

Occupational Adaptation: Study on Choice, Control, and Identity

Having presented studies of occupational adaptation from my experience and from the peer-reviewed literature, I turn now to a study completed in early 2017 in which we explored choice and control for people following spinal cord injury or brain injury (Stanley et al., 2018). The study employed a qualitative descriptive design: a design that is particularly suited for exploratory studies and a useful generic approach to qualitative research (Sandelowski, 2000). Ethical approval for the study was provided by the University of South Australia's Human Research Ethics Committee. The aim of the study was to generate a rich, in-depth understanding of the meaning of choice and control from the perspective of the person who had experienced major injury and his or her carers or family members. The reader may well ask at this point how this study of choice and control relates to a chapter about the experience of occupational adaptation, and at first glance they are two different topics; however, in talking about the role of choice and control in their recovery, the participants were describing occupational adaptation. So, although in this study occupational adaptation was not foregrounded, here I am going to bring the construct to the forefront while describing the role of choice and control and identity.

Participants were recruited with assistance from services that provide supports to people at home or during the transition period. Recruitment employed a maximum variation sampling approach with regard to variation in type and severity of injury and

Table 10-1

Choice and Control Study Participant Characteristics			
Participant	Overview	Age Bracket (years)	Sex
P1	ABI a year ago	40 to 49	M
P2	ABI 5 years ago	50 to 59	F
P3	ABI & SCI a year ago	50 to 59	M
P4	SCI 18 months ago	30 to 39	M
P5	Degenerative spinal cord condition, in a wheelchair since 2006	Did not wish to disclose	F
P6	ABI 18 months ago	30 to 39	F
P7	ABI 3 years ago	60 to 69	M
P8	ABI 3 years ago and again 1 year ago	50 to 59	M
P9	SCI a year ago	60 to 69	M
P10	ABI & SCI 3 years ago	40 to 49	M
C1	Carer for a person with SCI	50 to 59	F
C2	Carer for a person with SCI	30 to 39	F
C3	Carer for a person with SCI & ABI	50 to 59	F
C4	Carer for a person with ABI & SCI	40 to 49	F
Abbreviations: ABI, acquired brain injury; C, caregiver; F, female; M, male; P, participant; SCI, spinal cord injury.			

length of time since injury. Participants were included if they had transitioned from hospital and/or rehabilitation services between 12 months and 5 years ago, were able to recall their experience, and were able to undertake an oral interview.

We did a semi-structured, in-depth interview with each participant about his or her experience of transitioning back to the community and the role of choice and control. We analyzed the data generated from the interviews thematically, arriving at a rich description of participants' perspectives on choice and control and the role of reintegration to community.

Fourteen participants undertook in-depth interviews: two adults with a spinal cord injury, five adults with a brain injury, two adults with both a brain injury and spinal cord injury, an adult with a degenerative spinal cord condition, and four caregivers. The participants were between 30 and 66 years old, most participants with an injury were male, and all caregivers were female. Participant characteristics are presented in Table 10-1.

People wanted to have a sense of control in their own lives and commonly experienced a loss of control in the early stages after injury, with most (but not all) gradually regaining control. Loss of control was frustrating and depressing, and not all attempts to regain control were successful. People sought a level of control that was right for them, which for some was the choice to defer all decisions to someone else in order to cope. Control was understood by participants as a sense of being agentic through their own actions and expression of feelings and choices. Regaining control made participants feel good, calm, and more normal, whereas a lack of control increasing anxiety and anger.

> *Participant 6: When you have control, it just makes you ... it makes you feel better, it makes you be able to do things more easily, it makes you be able to think more clearly, makes you be able to deal with problems more easily as well.*

The participants' identity mediated control through their choices and their personal power. Following the injury, participants experienced significant loss of their old selves and a need to understand who they had become. In the process of getting to know their new abilities, they became selective about what was important for them to control. The growth in understanding was part of the process of learning to accept and adjust to their situation. They were then able to control the choices they made about how to self-regulate their routine and their occupations to accommodate what they could and wanted to control. The effect of a loss of control due to the actions of others generated a need for participants to exert personal power. Their attempts to exert personal power to gain control were not always successful, which had consequences for the relationships with those around them.

Identity as an Influence on Control

Following the brain injury or spinal cord injury (in some cases, participants had experienced both), participants experienced a major change in their identity. They grieved the loss of who they were and the occupations and friends who were part of their previous life. In recovery, they began exploring who they were going to become. They had to choose to take control of letting go, moving on, and creating a new identity as part of the natural trajectory of recovery from injury. Adjusting to the new or different set of capabilities and limits from the changed body was an ongoing process of discovery and involved making conscious choices about who they were going to be or wanted to become.

> *Participant 1: I guess one of the biggest things that I had to come to terms with was that old [name] may never come back ... You need to just ... just forget about it. What's new [name] going to look like and what are you going to do, or what steps do you need to take to get to whatever your new reality is going to be? I still don't know what that is, but I think from a conscious choice perspective that is something you have to decide.*

Being a worker was a strong part of many of the participants' previous identity. Returning to work was seen as a marker of progress and a return to normality for participants, but this was a difficult thing to control and achieve and was not always successful, requiring a revision of how they saw their identity.

> *Participant 3: The market had changed, the business had been going downhill, and I knew that I didn't have the mental faculties to go through the process of going and talking to clients, finding out what their needs were and then going and sourcing the products ...*

As participants reclaimed their identity or crafted a new identity, they found that being able to control things sustained them and enabled them to enjoy life created a sense of belonging to the community. This engagement in turn helped to establish the new identity, the new normal and a sense of feeling useful.

> *Participant 7: We have what they call the ... the blokes in the shed sort of thing. And one of the guys had a ... it was a fatal cancer of the brain and we went down there one day and trimmed up his big hedges that were out of control and stuff like that. It was a fun day. We did something positive and supported him, got something done for him. Us blokes had a good time doing it. It was good all around.*

Having choices was an important pathway to control. Participants could make choices about how they would respond to their situation, and some needed to build capacity and to find the mental tools to make the choice to accept and adjust to their situation.

Choices About Occupation

Participants recognized the need to make a choice to re-engage with the occupations of life. Choosing to keep occupied and to keep trying different occupations was important to giving participants their recovery and occupational adaptation. However, sometimes this required a need to exert personal power to control their environment, as illustrated in the following quote, where the participant needed a quiet environment in order to be successful in her occupational engagement.

> *Participant 2: ... So that I could keep going [to mosaic group] ... he wanted to put the radio on all the time, and it drove me nuts, I couldn't listen to that, listen to the people talk and make mosaics. So I started off by saying, "Look, it's bothering my hearing," but then I just kept switching it off all the time and they would say, "But we like listening to that." I'm going, "Well, I can't put up with it because I have a brain injury," and they went, "Oh, okay" and just turned it off.*

Establishing identity, having choices, and exerting agency to influence control were mediated by (1) having information and knowledge about their condition, care processes, and support systems; (2) the presence of powerful others who could assist and advocate for the person with injury; and (3) the approach used by health professionals.

Information and Knowledge as a Mediator of Identity, Choice, and Personal Power

Knowledge of health and social support systems were identified by participants as advantageous for helping them to know the right questions to ask and who and how to approach for support. Access to information was often difficult, or information was in a form that could not be easily understood in simple language with good explanations. Sometimes too much information was provided at once, and only provided once, making it difficult to comprehend and to remember.

> *Participant 7: So it was just too much information for me to process ...*

Access to information was an important aspect in the process of maintaining or reforming identity. Participants identified that part of their identity was as a sexual and/or intimate person, yet information on sexual health that supported the person's sense of being a sexual person was especially limited. Participants with brain injury found that discussions about sexual health were absent from their health care, with health professionals being too uncomfortable to broach the topic or assuming that people with a disability did not have a sexual identity. Helpful information about intimacy in relationships as well as sex was found by independently searching online; however, they would have preferred support and resources about these topics in discussions with health professionals.

Caregiver 2: Sexual health is a massive thing as well that I think is completely glossed over for a lot of people with disabilities … not just spinal cord injury, but for a lot of people with disabilities. They're not seen as sexual people anymore … I think that's a massive thing … like being able to control your sexual health.

Although choices were frequently limited, having a totally free choice was not necessarily helpful, particularly when participants did not have the required knowledge to make an informed and effective choice. When information was provided in a way that built the capacity of participants to make an informed choice, then it enabled participants to be in control and to self-manage. Information and education is also essential for support of the person with the injury. Participants suggested that this often gets forgotten.

Participant 7: … The information helps you, which helps you go down that path of choice. If you've got choice then that kind of leads on to control a bit because you've got a path that you can go down. So I think one leads into another.

In order for participants to exercise agency and make effective choices to exert control, they needed good information. Without adequate information about the topic being decided, participants felt vulnerable and powerless.

Participant 1: I think they talk about the knowledge being power … the couple of times where the couple of specialists did take the time to actually explain from A to Z, and having an understanding of what all that meant certainly made me feel a lot better, probably a little bit more in control, because I started to understand that it was okay to be like that or to feel that because in the past I didn't, because … I didn't know.

Powerful Others to Advocate and Support as a Mediator of Identity, Choice, and Personal Power

If participants were not able to express their own wishes for whatever reason, it was important for them to have an advocate who knew their personal preferences and values and could attend appointments with them to be assertive on their behalf. Having powerful support from others such as advocates, family members, or friends and peer support from those who have been in similar situations could make a difference to participants having a sense of control.

The Approach Used by Health Professionals as a Mediator of Identity, Choice, and Personal Power

Little credit was given to participants for knowledge of their own body and condition. Professionals were perceived to know what they were doing but did not always listen and came with assumptions about what was right for people without knowing the individual person. It was critical for participants to feel they had a voice and were heard during interactions with professionals. A loss of voice was associated with a potential loss of control and loss of identity and potentially delayed the process of occupational adaptation.

> *Participant 8: I hate the feeling of being trapped, and I wanted to go for a walk every day, and I ended up going for a walk regardless of what they said. Every time I went out, I had to promise that I would be back … just being questioned all the time. I know they've got responsibility for me and they need to know where I am, but to be able to sign in and sign out and say where I'm going to be would have been really nice rather than held under suspicion all the time.*

Participants often felt that their identity was reduced to "an image on a screen or a blood test result" and that they were given generic care that was not personalized or did not incorporate an understanding of who they were as a person. Participants described approaches that created dependent identities rather than building their capacity and independence, such as being told that if they had questions or concerns they should contact the health professionals rather than being empowered with knowledge about information and resources they could independently find and use. Health professionals were described as assuming the expert role, using jargon, and taking over. It seems self-evident that if health professionals took a more enabling approach to information giving and capacity building, the process of occupational adaptation would be enhanced.

> *Participant 6: … And you're not allowing me to get on with what I know I can do independently, and you're not talking to me like a normal human being either.*

When health professionals removed participant choice and took a rigid approach to making decisions on their behalf, participants began to foster a distrust of them and the system in general. There were numerous stories of mismanagement of medications and health care and a reliance on reasoning related to the person's condition rather taking a person-centred approach.

Participants perceived that health professionals exerted significant power over them, which affected their recovery and their feelings of control. It was important to participants to retain hope for a better future, and having goals and plans were a means of feeling in control. In contrast, participants perceived that hope for complete recovery was often viewed by health professionals as unrealistic and not helpful, and they provided many examples of their hope for future recovery being squashed by professionals.

> *Participant 8: And then the neurologist—I hate neurologists—she told me I would never, ever work again in any capacity. And that didn't make me feel too good at all … All my hobbies and activities and she said, "Forget everything. You can't do any of that; you're too active. Find more sedate things to do." And yeah, that was pretty devastating, but anyway … I found another neurologist.*

One participant was upset and perceived that he was "told off" by the exercise physiologist for over-exercising when he chose to exceed the number of required repetitions for an exercise because he felt he knew his body and it was okay. The participant's entire focus was on rehabilitation and recovery, and he just wanted to work harder to get better. His identity was created around being in rehabilitation and doing exercise. From reading the transcript and seeing the importance of identity in the analysis of findings, it was apparent that this participant had little else to focus on in his life. If he could find meaningful occupations to engage in, he could have begun the reclaiming of his identity with the new set of capacities instead of being stuck in the stage of rehabilitation several years after injury and feeling at the mercy of the health professionals for making decisions in his life.

In stark contrast, there were approaches from health professionals that participants found capacity building as empowering, and they were able to make some recommendations about what approaches they preferred to support control over their recovery. These included health professionals emphasizing what they could do and what they may be able to try within their new capabilities, as well as taking an interest in building their resources for coping.

> Participant 5: Ask them [injured people] what they think and see if you can help them in any way ... ask them how they're going and everything like that.

PULLING THE COMMON THREADS TOGETHER

From all of the studies presented in this chapter, it is evident that there is a tight nexus between occupational identity and occupational adaptation. It has led me to think about the merging of Schultz and Schkade's (1997) early work on occupational adaptation, with the mismatch between the demands of the occupation, the environment, and the capacities of the person, with Kielhofner's (2008) conceptualization of occupational adaptation, which includes occupational identity. Occupational adaptation is not a linear process, but rather an iterative, dynamic process of interplay between occupational engagement and occupational identity.

The occupational adaptation process begins with a realization that the anticipated occupational future may no longer be possible. There is an associated period of grief as that imagined future is discarded and eventually replaced with a reimagined future, which more closely reflects the person's capacity. Engaging in novel and familiar occupations is the medium through which people test out their capacities to find the right fit. They need to explore which occupations are no longer able to be part of their occupational repertoire and thus no longer a part of how they identify as an occupational being. They also need to try new occupations or bring forward occupations that they may have engaged in in the past to test the fit with current capacity or to explore occupational engagement to achieve mastery. The new occupational engagement enables the person to claim or reclaim their occupational identity and thus achieve occupational adaptation. There is acceptance of a new reality that resonates with the new or reclaimed occupational identity.

From the studies reviewed here, along with other studies, it is evident that the conceptual development of occupational adaptation is moving toward a formal theory. It can be developed further, as Nayar and Stanley (2014) have suggested, by conducting more studies of different transitions and by taking a grounded theory approach to study process. The majority of published studies, or the most developed areas, have been with groups that occupational therapists have a lot of contact with, such as aging people or people following a stroke or brain injury. In addition, occupational scientists have focussed on migration. Other parts of the life span and other transitions that might not be typically associated with disability also warrant investigation. As in many areas of research within occupational therapy and occupational science, most studies emanate from North America and Australasia, and there is little written from parts of the world in different contexts or that have a more collectivist view of the world.

RETURNING TO DANIEL AND BEULAH

At the start to this chapter, I recounted the stories of Daniel, who had been retrenched, and Beulah, whose husband had died. Taking a closer look at each of these stories, it is possible to anticipate the reactions to both situations and how that impacts on their occupational engagement (Table 10-2). Now, taking the information presented in this chapter, it is possible to see how both Daniel and Beulah could achieve occupational adaptation through occupation. In the process, they would develop a new occupational identity of being resilient despite the challenges of job loss or loss of a life partner.

The challenges presented in the stories of Daniel and Beulah are just two of the many challenging transitions that occur in life but point to the key role that occupational engagement plays in health and well-being. For both transitions, there is the initial experience of shock and loss; the associated emotional reactions of grief, fear, and anger; and major occupational disruption. In time, the people begin to develop new routines, try new occupations, or re-engage with previous occupations. They begin to reshape their identities as someone who is currently not a worker but between jobs or looking for work, or as someone who is now without a partner. It is through occupational engagement that the new identity is shaped and occupational adaptation occurs.

IMPLICATIONS

The findings point to the need for occupational therapists to use their expertise in occupation when working with clients. Drawing on the skills in occupational analysis, therapists can find the just-right challenge so that clients can test the limits of their capacities and achieve or work toward mastery. Although the focus of therapy is usually on enabling occupational performance, it is evident that there also needs to be a focus on the client's occupational identity and occupational adaptation. Understanding who the client is and his or her values and priorities becomes even more important in order to enable occupational adaptation. A thorough occupational history will enable the occupational therapist to gain that understanding.

Table 10-2

Occupational Adaptation for Daniel and Beulah				
Name	What Would the Person Be Experiencing?	What Changes Would Occur in Their Life?	What Stages Might Be Involved in the Transition to the New Life?	How Would the Person Manage/ Negotiate the Transition?
Daniel	Loss, resignation, loss of self-worth, fear, anticipation, excitement, challenge to masculinity	Loss of worker role, change in financial status, change in identity, no work structure, new freedom	Honeymoon period that is like a holiday, boredom, new routines	Fill time with time killers or engaging occupations, new routine, home maintenance and domestic tasks, volunteering, job seeking
Beulah	Grief, loss, loss of appetite, loss of purpose, loneliness	Live alone after years of sharing her life and home, loss of company, loss of shared routines, change in roles	Loss, anger, despair, in time readjusting and re-engaging, trying new occupations, the new life as a single person	Organize for others to do some occupations (e.g. gardening, driving). Take on roles that Silas used to do and related occupations; re-engage socially, possibly with new occupations or previously meaningful ones

I often hear from therapists that they don't have time to collect a thorough occupational history; however, I argue that the time taken to gain that in-depth understanding of the person is extremely worthwhile in building rapport and gaining the engagement of the client in therapy, which will lead to better and more sustainable outcomes. Indeed, it is best practice, and the focus on occupational engagement is the valuable contribution that occupational therapists bring to the lives of clients that no other health professional has the expertise to do. Occupational therapists need to own their expertise, champion it, and use its power.

ADVANCING THE KNOWLEDGE ON OCCUPATIONAL ADAPTATION

In this chapter, I have drawn on a number of primary and secondary studies of occupational adaptation from a range of occupational transitions. Those transitions have included occupational disruption from brain injury or stroke, becoming a parent to a pre-term infant, being a caregiver, migrating, and aging. The findings across all of the studies show that occupational identity has a tight nexus with occupational adaptation and that occupational engagement is the medium to occupational adaptation for health and well-being. I have highlighted the need for more studies of other occupational transitions and the gap in knowledge from a variety of cultural groups. I have also highlighted the importance of taking the knowledge about occupational adaptation and applying in occupational therapy practice by enabling people to re-engage in occupations or find new meaningful occupations in order to test the limit of capacities and to reclaim or reshape their occupational identity.

SUMMARY AND IMPLICATIONS

- Occupational adaptation is precipitated by a mismatch between the demands of an occupation, the environment, and the capacities of the person.
- People who have experienced an occupational disruption need to reclaim their occupational identity.
- Engagement in occupation is the medium for testing the limits of capacity and achieving mastery, and therefore the mechanism for occupational adaptation.
- Occupational adaptation is a process.
- A greater focus on occupational identity is warranted in practice.

REFERENCES

Beck, B., Bray, J., Cameron, P., Cooper, D. J., & Gabbe, B. (2016). Trends in severe traumatic brain injury in Victoria, 2006-2014. *Medical Journal of Australia*, *204*(11), 407. doi:10.5694/mja15.01369

Eaves, Y. D. (2001). A synthesis technique for grounded theory data analysis. *Journal of Advanced Nursing*, *35*(5), 654-663. doi:10.1046/j.1365-2648.2001.01897.x

Gibbs, D., Boshoff, K., & Stanley, M. (2015). Becoming the parent of a preterm infant: A meta-ethnographic synthesis. *British Journal of Occupational Therapy*, *78*(8), 475-487. doi:10.1177/0308022615586799

Gibbs, D., Boshoff, K., & Stanley, M. (2016). The acquisition of parenting occupations in neonatal intensive care: A preliminary perspective. *Canadian Journal of Occupational Therapy*, *83*(2), 91-102. doi:10.1177/0008417415625421

Hillier, S., Hillier, J., & Metzer, J. (1997). Epidemiology of traumatic brain injury in South Australia. *Brain Injury*, *11*(9), 649-659.

Kielhofner, G. (2008). *Model of human occupation: Theory and application* (4th ed.). Baltimore, MD: Lippincott Williams & Wilkins.

McDougall, C., Buchanan, A., & Peterson, S. (2014). Understanding primary carers' occupational adaptation and engagement. *Australian Occupational Therapy Journal*, *61*, 83-91. doi:10.1111/1440-1630.12076

Nayar, S., & Stanley, M. (2014). Occupational adaptation as a social process in everyday life. *Journal of Occupational Science, 22*(1), 26-38. doi:10.1080/14427591.2014.882251

Parsons, L., & Stanley, M. (2008). The lived experience of occupational adaptation following acquired brain injury for people living in a rural area. *Australian Occupational Therapy Journal, 55*, 231-238. doi:10.1111/j.1440-1630.2008.00753.x

Sandelowski, M. (2000). Whatever happened to qualitative description? *Research in Nursing and Health, 23*, 334-340.

Schatzman, L. (1991). Dimensional analysis: Notes on an alternative approach to the grounding of theory in qualitative research. In D. R. Maines (Ed.), *Social organization and social process* (pp. 303-314). New York, NY: Aldine De Gruyter.

Schultz, S., & Schkade, J. (1997). Adaptation. In C. H. Christiansen & C. Baum (Eds.), *Occupational therapy: Enabling function and well-being* (pp. 458-481). Thorofare, NJ: SLACK Incorporated.

Soeker, M. S. (2011). Occupational adaptation: A return to work perspective of persons with mild to moderate brain injury in South Africa. *Journal of Occupational Science, 17*(1), 81-91. doi:10.1080/144275 91.2011.554155

Stanley, M. (2009). *Older people's understanding of well-being.* Saarbrucken, Germany: VDM Verdlag.

Stanley, M., Mackintosh, S., van Kessell, G., Fryer, C., Murray, C., & Hillier, S. (2018). *Connections between choice, control and occupational identity for people with spinal cord or brain injury.* Paper presented at the 2018 World Federation of Occupational Therapists Congress, Cape Town, South Africa. Abstract retrieved from http://www.wfotcongress.org/downloads/abstracts/SE%2042/Connections%20between%20choice.pdf

Walder, K., & Molineux, M. (2017). Occupational adaptation and identity reconstruction: A groundedtheory synthesis of qualitative studies exploring adults' experiences of adjustment to chronic disease, major illness or injury. *Journal of Occupational Science, 24*(2), 225-243. doi:10.1080/14427591.2016. 1269240

Wells, S. A. (2015). Occupational deprivation or occupational adaptation of Mexican Americans on renal dialysis. *Occupational Therapy International, 22*, 174-182. doi:10.1002/oti.1394

Williams, S., & Murray, C. (2013). The lived experience of older adults' occupational adaptation following a stroke. *Australian Occupational Therapy Journal, 60*(1), 39-47. doi:10.1111/1440-1630.12004

Financial Disclosures

Dr. Rebecca M. Aldrich has no financial or proprietary interest in the materials presented herein.

Dr. Mary Frances Baxter has no financial or proprietary interest in the materials presented herein.

Dr. Angela K. Boisselle has no financial or proprietary interest in the materials presented herein.

Dr. Patricia Bowyer is lead author of the *Short Child Occupational Profile*, published and sold by the University of Illinois Chicago MOHO Clearinghouse. She received royalties for the assessment.

Dr. Elaina DaLomba has no financial or proprietary interest in the materials presented herein.

Dr. Evan E. Dean has no financial or proprietary interest in the materials presented herein.

Dr. Katherine Dimitropoulou has no financial or proprietary interest in the materials presented herein.

Dr. Winifred Dunn is author of *Sensory Profiles*, published and sold by Pearson. She received honoraria for the assessment.

Dr. Lorrie George-Paschal has no financial or proprietary interest in the materials presented herein.

Dr. Lenin C. Grajo has no financial or proprietary interest in the materials presented herein.

Dr. Kendra Heatwole Shank has no financial or proprietary interest in the materials presented herein.

Dr. Lauren Little has no financial or proprietary interest in the materials presented herein.

Dr. Dawn M. Nilsen has no financial or proprietary interest in the materials presented herein.

Dr. Sally W. Schultz has no financial or proprietary interest in the materials presented herein.

Dr. Mandy Stanley was part of a study that was financially supported by the Lifetime Support Authority.

Dr. Anna Wallisch has no financial or proprietary interest in the materials presented herein.

Index

action observation, 51–52
activity, in ICF model, 86, 89, 165
adaptation, construct of, xix, 4
adaptation gestalt, 90–91
adaptive capacity, 25–27, 53, 92–94, 97, 100–101
adaptive response mechanism, 62, 91
adaptive responses, 42, 62, 182
    definition of, 91
    occupational science perspectives on, 163–164
    occupations as central to eliciting, 99–100
    press for mastery, related to, 91–92
    sensory processing and, 124–125, 129–132
adapt/modify intervention strategy, 149
advocacy, 144, 186
aging, 71–72, 181–182
allocation of occupations, 181–182
allostasis, 66
allostatic load, 66
alter intervention strategy, 148–149
American Occupational Therapy Association (AOTA), 6, 85–86, 88, 89, 161
amygdala, 63, 64
anterior cingulate cortex, 64
apoptosis, 40–41
assessments. *See* measures of occupational participation
avoiding (sensory processing pattern), 126–127, 134–135
awareness, promotion of, 74

basal ganglia, 63
BAT (bilateral training), 49–50
becoming, concept of, 5, 13
behavioral intervention studies, 74
bilateral training (BAT), 49–50
biological stressors, 72–73
body functions and body structures, in ICF model, 86, 88
brain injury, lived experience of, 177–178
brain structures and circuits, 62–64

caregiving for pre-term infants, lived experience of, 178–179
catastrophic change, 116–117
change
    in Model of Human Occupation (MOHO), 116–117
    occupational science perspectives on, 164–165, 168
    as theme in scoping study, 12
choice, and adaptive capacity, 26
choice, in OA-guided intervention, 98–99
choice and control study, 182–188
CIMT (constraint-induced movement therapy), 45, 49, 52–53
client as agent of change, 98–99
client factors, in Occupational Therapy Practice Framework, 86, 88
client-centered approach, 24, 97–99, 144, 145, 165
coaching, use of sensory processing knowledge in, 133

cognitive control, 71
cognitive reframing, 167
cognitive reserve, model of, 71–72
cognitive vs physical effort, 66
communication and interaction skills, 112
Community of Practice, 101
compensatory masquerade, 44
constraint-induced movement therapy (CIMT), 49, 52–53
construct of adaptation. *See* occupational adaptation, construct of
contexts, in Occupational Therapy Practice Framework, 86, 88
control, perceived, 181–182
control of health process, 74
control study. *See* choice and control study
convergence, 39
cortisol, 67
cost-benefit ratio, 65–66
create intervention strategy, 149–150
cross-modal reassignment (cross-modal plasticity), 42–43
cultural environment, 75, 115, 146
cultural spaces, navigating, 180–181
culturally relevant practice, 95–96
cumulative repertoire, 11

demand for mastery, 88, 89
dendritic spines, 38
desire for mastery, 88, 89
desired sense of self, 12–13
developmental changes, 40–41, 70–73, 131–132
dimensions of doing, 106, 111–113
Distinct Value statement, 6
divergence, 39
doing, dimensions of, 111–113
dopamine network, 64–66
dysadaptive responses, 91–92. *See also* occupational dysadaptation

Ecology of Human Performance (EHP), 141–155
    basic assumptions, 143–145
    core constructs, 145–147
    occupational adaptation, view of, 142, 154
    therapeutic intervention
        case study, 150–154
        common language phrases for, 148
        strategies, 147–150
effective participation, 22, 93–94, 97
efficiency, 22, 93–94, 97
emotions related to need (or demand) for adaptation, 26

empowerment of client as agent of change, 98–99
end-stage renal disease, lived experience of, 177–178
engagement. *See* occupational engagemenet
environment, 13
    adaptive capacity and, 26
    demands of, 4, 26
    in Ecology of Human Performance (EHP) Model, 143–147, 151–153
    lived experience of occupational adaptation and, 178–179, 181, 185
    in Model of Human Occupation (MOHO), 110, 115
    neurobiological processes and, 70–71, 72, 74–75
    in Occupational Adaptation (OA) model, 86, 88, 99–100
    occupational science perspectives on, 162–165, 168
    in Sensory Processing Model, 124, 128, 131, 133–134
    as theme in scoping study, 11
environmental factors, in ICF model, 86, 88
environments, in Occupational Therapy Practice Framework, 86, 88
epigenetic factors, 68, 72
establish/restore intervention strategy, 148

focal-task specific dystonia (FTSD), 44
functional plasticity at the modular level, 42–44

general systems theory, 161–162
genetic factors, 71, 72, 73, 131
goal-directed actions, 45, 61–62, 69, 71, 112
goals, self-initiated, 70, 98–99
grounded theory studies, 180–182

habits, 109
habituation, 109–110
health, access to information about, 185–186
health, awareness and control of, 74
health professionals, approach used by, 187–188
heterosynaptic plasticity, 41
holistic assessment, 96–97
homeostasis, definition of, 66
homeostasis, regulation of, 64
homeostatic state, and exposure to stress, 73
homologous area adaptation, 42
homosynaptic plasticity, 41
hormones, 64–69, 73
hyper-responsiveness, 127

hypo-responsiveness, 126–127
hypothalamus-pituitary-adrenal (HPA) axis,
    68–69

incremental change, 116
independence, 144–145, 181–182, 187
information, access to, 185–186
instruments. *See* measures of occupational
    participation
intention, 61, 69, 71
interest, in Model of Human Occupation, 109
internalized roles, 109–110
International Classification of Functioning,
    Disability and Health (ICF), 86, 88–89,
    165–166

knowledge of health and support systems,
    185–186

life transitions, as theme in literature, 12
"lived body," 110
lived experience of occupational adaptation, 10,
    14, 175–192
    following brain injury, stroke, and end-stage
        renal disease, 177–178
    grounded theory studies, 180–182
    occupational adaptation, definition of, 13, 175
    occupational identity and, 180–182,
        184–190
    parenting and caregiving of pre-term infants,
        178–179
    performance capacity and, 110
    studies, conclusions based on, 188–189
    study on choice and control, 182–188
long-term depression (LTD), 41
long-term potentiation (LTP), 41

maladaptive neural responses, 44, 72–73
map expansion, 43–44
mastery, sense of, 12–13, 74, 88. *See also* press
    for mastery; relative mastery
meaningful occupation, 4, 11, 26
measures of occupational participation, 19–31,
    117–118
    adaptive capacity, 25–27, 92–94, 97,
        100–101
    gap in literature on, 14
    holistic assessments, 96–97
    instrument development studies, 11, 14
    occupational identity and occupational
        competence, 23–25
    relative mastery, 20–23, 92–94, 97, 100–101

memory formation, 11, 41
mental practice, 50
mirror therapy, 51
Model of Human Occupation (MOHO), 10,
    105–121
    assessment tools, 14, 24–25, 117–118
    conceptual beginnings, 107
    constructs of, 108–111
    dimensions of doing, 111–113
    occupational adaptation and, 112–113
        change, types of, 116–117
        definition of, 5, 23, 115
        environment as factor in, 115
        evidence for, 117, 119
        life phases, 115
        manifested through occupational identity
            and occupational competence, 23–25,
            113–114, 119
modify/adapt intervention strategy, 149
modular neuroplasticity, 42–44
motivation, 61, 64–66, 69, 71, 74
motor skill learning, 43–44, 45–53
motor skills, and dimensions of doing, 112–113
motor skills, definition of, 112

natural vs contrived contexts, 99–100, 143–144
neural basis of adaptation. *See also*
    neuroplasticity
    adaptive capacity and, 25
    brain, midsagittal view of, 62
    brain structures and circuits, 62–64
    children vs adults, 71
    creating conditions for recovery, 73–75
    developmental changes, 40–41, 70–73
    dopamine network, 64–66
    goal-directed behavior, 45, 61–62, 69, 71
    intention and, 61, 69, 71
    motivation and, 61, 64–66, 69, 71, 74
    neurons and neuronal communication,
        36–39, 61–62
    resilience and, 61, 64, 66–69, 74, 75
    sensory processing and, 126, 131–132
    stress, impact of, 72–75
    stress neurochemical networks, 66–69
neuronal circuits, 38–39, 61–62
neuronal communication, 37
neuronal membrane, 37–38
neurons, function and structure of, 36–38, 61–62
neurons, pruning of (apoptosis), 40, 73
neuropeptide Y, 67
neuroplasticity, 60
    definition of, 36

factors contributing to, 70–72
maladaptive, 44, 72–73
maladaptive, reversal of, 50–51
recovery of function and, 45
   case study, 52–53
   engagement in novel activities, 50–53
   intervention studies, 46–48
   task-oriented training interventions, 45,
     49–50, 52–53
types of, 39–44
neuroscience. *See* neural basis of adaptation;
   neuroplasticity
neurotransmitters, 38, 64–69

occupational activities, 99
occupational adaptation, construct of, 189
   foundational viewpoints, xix
   lack of uniform definition of, 4, 13–14
   as measure of occupational participation,
     19–31
   as process and outcome, 5–6, 10, 13–14
   scoping review of literature, 7–16
     definitions and themes from, 10–13
     frequency analysis, 9
     gaps in evidence and research, 13–14
     results, 8–10
     search strategy and selection process, 8
   use in practice, 6–7, 10
Occupational Adaptation (OA) model, 83–104
   adaptive capacity, 25–27, 53, 92–94, 97,
     100–101
   approximation of concepts with Framework
     and ICF language, 86, 88–89
   assessments, 14, 22–23, 25, 92–94, 96–97
   case studies, 87, 95
   client as agent of change, 98–99
   clinical application of, 6–7, 101
   as conceptual model, 95–96
   core principles of, 83
   internal normative process, 87–94
   intervention process, 94–101
   occupational adaptation, definition of, 5, 87,
     163–164
   occupational environment and, 88, 99–100
   occupational participation and, 88–89
   occupational roles, 89, 92, 97–98
   occupations as central to adaptive responses,
     99–100
   person and person systems, 88, 90–91, 99
   press for mastery, 89–92
     adaptation gestalt, 90–91
     adaptive and dysadaptive responses, 91–92

     calibration of, 89–90
     definition of, 89
     visual analysis of, 92
   process and outcome in, 5–6
   process illustration, 85
   reconceptualization, rationale for, 84–85
   relative mastery, 6, 20–23, 92–94, 97,
     100–101
   scoping review of literature and, 10, 14
   state and process aspect of, 85–87
occupational adaptiveness, 87, 92–94, 97,
   100–101, 103
occupational challenges, 89–90, 92
occupational choices, 169, 182–188
occupational competence, 12–13, 23–25, 114, 119
occupational consciousness, 169
occupational demands, 86, 89
occupational dysadaptation, 26, 89, 92, 94–95, 99
occupational engagement, 6, 11, 13, 188
occupational environment, 11, 13, 86, 88, 99–100
occupational form, 111
occupational history, 189–190
occupational identity
   lived experience of occupational adaptation
     and, 180–182, 184–190
   in Model of Human Occupation (MOHO),
     23–25, 107, 113–114, 119
   occupational science research on, 166
   as theme in scoping study, 12–13
occupational justice, 168–169
occupational participation
   in Model of Human Occupation (MOHO),
     111–113
   occupational adaptation as measure of, 19–31
   occupational adaptation as outcome of, 5–6,
     13–14
   in Occupational Adaptation (OA) model, 86,
     88–89
   occupational justice and, 168–169
   occupational science perspectives on,
     165–167
   in Sensory Processing Model, 124–125,
     129–130, 132, 135
occupational performance, 23, 133
   in Ecology of Human Performance (EHP)
     Model, 146–147, 154
   lived experience of occupational adaptation,
     181–182
   in Model of Human Occupation (MOHO),
     111–113
   occupational science perspectives on, 165–166
occupational profile, 97, 117

occupational readiness, 99
occupational repertoire, 11
occupational responses, 90–92
occupational roles, 89, 92, 97–98
occupational science, 10, 159–174
    development of concepts
        adaptation, 5, 160, 163–165, 168
        occupation, 161–163, 168
        occupational justice, 168–169
        participation, 165–168
    origins and advances of discipline, 160–161
occupational skills, 112–113
occupational therapist, role of, 6, 98–99, 102
Occupational Therapy Practice Framework, 6,
    86, 88, 89
occupational well-being, 181–182
occupation-based programming, 75
occupations
    lived experience of occupational adaptation
        and, 177–178, 180–182, 185
    as means and end of therapy, xv–xvi
    in Occupational Adaptation (OA) model, 86,
        88–89, 99–100
    occupational science perspectives on, 161–163
    in Occupational Therapy Practice
        Framework, 86, 89
    scoping study themes and, 11
outcome, occupational adaptation as, 5–6, 10,
    13–14
outcome measurement. *See* measures of
    occupational participation

parenting pre-term infants, lived experience of,
    178–179
parent-mediated interventions, use of sensory
    processing knowledge in, 133
participation, in ICF model, 86, 89, 165–166
perceived control, 181–182
performance capacity, 110
performance patterns, 88
performance range, 146–147
performance skills, 86, 88
person (or person factors)
    adaptive capacity and, 26–27
    in Ecology of Human Performance (EHP)
        Model, 143, 145–147, 150–152
    in Model of Human Occupation (MOHO),
        108–111
    in Occupational Adaptation (OA) model, 86,
        88, 90–91, 99
    in Sensory Processing Model, 124–125
personal causation, 108

phasic mode, 65
Philosophical Base of Occupational Therapy,
    6, 85
physical environment, 100, 146
physical vs cognitive effort, 66
place integration, 164–165
prefrontal cortex, 62–63
press for mastery, 89–92
    adaptation gestalt, 90–91
    adaptive and dysadaptive responses, 91–92
    calibration of, 89–90
    definition of, 89
    visual analysis of, 92
pre-term infants, parenting of, 178–179
prevent intervention strategy, 149
process, occupational adaptation as, 5, 10,
    13–14, 85–87
process skills, 112
psychological stressors, 72–73
purpose, sense of, 74

registration (sensory processing pattern),
    126–127, 134–135
regulation of homeostasis, 64
relational perspectives, 167
relative mastery, 6, 20–23, 92–94, 97, 100–101
repetitive activity, 43–44, 49–50
resilience, 61, 64, 66–69, 74, 75
restore/establish intervention strategy, 148
reward processing, 64–65
role demands or expectations, 89, 92, 100
role-focused approach, 97–98
roles, in Model of Human Occupation, 109–110

satisfaction, 11, 22, 93–94, 97
scoping review of literature, 7–16
    definitions and themes from, 10–13
    frequency analysis, 9
    gaps in evidence and research, 13–14
    limitations, 14
    results, 8–10
    search strategy and selection process, 8
seeking (sensory processing pattern), 126–127,
    134–135
self, desired sense of, 12–13
self-awareness, 74
self-belief, 177
self-determination, 144
self-initiated goals, 70, 98–99
sensitivity (sensory processing pattern), 126–127,
    134–135
sensory features, 125

Sensory Processing, 123–140
  adaptive responses and, 124–125, 129–132
  biological and neural mechanisms, 131–132
  contemporary models of, 126–127
  in context of occupational adaptation,
      124–125
  definition of, 124
  evidence related to adaptation and, 129–135
  historical perspectives, 126
  interventions to support occupational
      adaptation and, 132–135
    collaborating with families, 133
    environment-focused, 133–134
    examples of strategies to improve
        participation, 135
    structures for organizing knowledge,
        127–129
  terminology, 125
sensory processing differences, 125
Sensory Processing Framework, 126–127
serotonin receptors (5-HT), 67
shaping, in behavioral conditioning, 49
shaping self, 180–181
social contexts, 100, 146, 162, 164–167, 178
social supports, 26, 74–75
specifications, 61
spiritual supports, 75
state, in Occupational Adaptation (OA) model,
    85–87
stress, impact of, 72–75

stress neurochemical networks, 66–69
stroke, lived experience of, 177–178
support systems, 26, 74–75
synapses, 38
synaptic cleft, 38
synaptic plasticity, 41–42
synaptic transmission, 38

task, in Ecology of Human Performance (EHP)
    Model, 146–147, 150–152
task-oriented training interventions, 45, 49–50,
    52–53
tonic mode, 65
trading off, 181–182
transactional process/perspectives, xix, 36
  in Ecology of Human Performance (EHP)
      Model, 143
  as factor in adaptive capacity, 26
  lived experience of occupational adaptation,
      178–179, 181
  occupational science perspectives on, 162
  press for mastery and, 89
  as theme in scoping study, 11
transformational change, 116

value, in Model of Human Occupation, 109
value changes, 182
virtual reality (VR), 52–53
volition, 26, 108–109